Science *and* Logic *in* Medical Diagnosis

IN DEFENSE OF INDIVIDUAL PATIENTS

Lee Forstrom

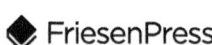
FriesenPress

Suite 300 - 990 Fort St
Victoria, BC, V8V 3K2
Canada

www.friesenpress.com

Copyright © 2020 by Lee Forstrom
First Edition — 2020

All rights reserved.

No part of this publication may be reproduced in any form, or by any means, electronic or mechanical, including photocopying, recording, or any information browsing, storage, or retrieval system, without permission in writing from FriesenPress.

ISBN
978-1-5255-5333-2 (Hardcover)
978-1-5255-5334-9 (Paperback)
978-1-5255-5335-6 (eBook)

1. MEDICAL, CLINICAL MEDICINE

Distributed to the trade by The Ingram Book Company

Acknowledgements

This manuscript is the outcome of my own work and includes no material resulting from work done in collaboration. Indebtedness is expressed, however, to the many mentors and friends who have offered advice and criticism helpful in its preparation. Special thanks in this regard are due to Professor Mary Hesse of the University of Cambridge (Philosophy) and to Professor Paul Holmer of the Universities of Minnesota and Yale (Philosophy). Many others have my gratitude, including Professor Richard Braithwaite of University of Cambridge (Philosophy), and other friends and colleagues in medicine. Financial assistance for part of early work from the United States National Institutes of Health Fellowship (1-F03-GM55985-01). National Institute of General Medical Sciences is also gratefully acknowledged. Above all, gratitude is expressed for the unfaltering support and encouragement of my family.

TABLE OF CONTENTS

INTRODUCTION

Perspectives

The object of this book is the diagnostic process in clinical medicine. Particular attention will be devoted to the internal logic of this process as it is utilized by practicing physicians. Most of the examples chosen for purposes of illustration are from the fields of medicine with which I am most familiar: internal medicine and nuclear medicine. However, I believe the logical structure of the diagnostic process to be similar in most other branches of medicine. At least some exceptions will be discussed.

Important as clinical medicine has been and is to society, few human activities are less understood, or subject to opinions more obscured by prejudice, myth, and misconception. The reasons for this are undoubtedly complex, but likely relate to the highly emotional and serious nature of the contacts between medicine and individual lives. Another reason may be the recent period of rapid growth and development in medical science and technology. Yet another reason must be the relative failure of physicians and philosophers to examine the methodological and ethical issues, among others, in medicine. Consideration of the diagnostic process, a critical part of medical decision-making, provides a focus from which it is hoped some light may be shed on other issues concerning the physician's status as scientist and healer. A fuller and more widespread understanding of this status would have useful social, legal, and educational ramifications. Certain of these will be taken up in later sections. However, two introductory propositions concerning the physician's status will be expressed and briefly discussed.

Behind misunderstanding of the physician's work is the apparent belief that medical diagnoses are, or should be, fairly obvious to the physician, either because they are somehow intrinsically clear to any properly trained observer or because the physician possesses some extraordinary powers of perceiving the hidden. The latter supposition, rooted perhaps in wish and magic, is quite plainly false. The former supposition simply misconstrues the nature of modern diagnostic concepts. Most diagnoses are now arrived at not by simple inspection, but by a more or less complex process combining examination, inference, testing, more inference, and so on. This process depends on common (fallible) scientific methods. The resulting diagnosis is usually tentative and (in a sense to be discussed) only "probable." The best diagnostician will therefore be wrong part of the time,[1] and a wrong diagnosis does not imply a mistake in his judgement, although these may also occur. Diagnostic success is at best a frequent thing, and such success will depend largely on the physician's knowledge, experience, and thoroughness of her/his examination, testing, and reasoning. This simple fact, of obvious economic and legal importance as well as patient satisfaction, is often ignored.[2] Clearly, discussion in medical ethics should rest on an understanding of medical methods.

Such situations may develop, for example, in the physician's examinations and tests, which are (with or without explanation) not related in the patient's mind to her/his symptoms or present disease. How often is there no self-diagnosis? Again, the physician may from available evidence properly suspect a disease that may be serious but in fact is not present. The tests she/he performs with "negative" outcomes ordinarily involve expense, discomfort, and some risk to the patient. The frequency in which this occurs trends upward with the seriousness of the suspected disease, and with the thoroughness of the physician. Performance of medical exams, tests, and procedures with negative outcomes may thus be seen as unnecessary. Generally, this idea rests on an overly simple view of medical diagnosis, stemming from misconceptions about the physician's methods, motives, and medical ethics. Given the prevailing (and presumably permanent) imperfect state of knowledge, however, negative diagnostic outcomes can be properly understood as an unavoidable aspect of medical standards. They will be seen to play an important role in the diagnostic process.

Linking and placing topics

Again, this manuscript is to examine and compare approaches to finding causes of sickness or injury (etc.) in a human patient, such that the cause can be treated correctly and promptly. Other issues include ethical concern for the patient's individual history, wishes, and nuances, and the growing use of genetics. The clinician may be short on time and the patient short on funds or time, but most clinicians and patients alike should prefer best available medical diagnosis. Two dominant and controversial approaches ("models") will be compared, along with a few asides.

In Western nations for at least a century or so, a scientific model has been common among professional clinicians for finding the cause of a sickness. This is not to say that similar approaches to disease had not been used much earlier. Nonetheless, Dr. Richard Cabot (1868 – 1939) at MGH (Boston) crossed a threshold in forming a diagnostic model based on causes of sickness. This was called "differential-diagnosis," and potential causes are called "hypotheses." Both remain the same now, but quite a lot has changed, as explained in the following chapters (specifically 3-7).

In this model, the sickness—signs and symptoms as "manifestations"—must connect to one or more of potential causes, and this has been called "deductive" or "inductive," terms from logical methods. Perhaps it was seen to fit with the fictional detective Sherlock Holmes and his deductive reasoning, created by physician Sir Arthur Conan Doyle (Scotland, 1859-1930). Thus, Cabot's model was coined "hypothetico-deductive," and it continues in medical usage today. Clinicians know, however, that deductive reasoning is not enough for all diagnoses. Reasoning with probabilities is usually needed.

Next came Carl G. Hempel (British, 1905-1997), an eminent philosopher of science who advocated a "covering-law" model for explanation and prediction in science. He created a "deductive-nomological" model, and another form the "inductive-statistical" model. These models were designed for objective probabilities, but can be equally used with subjective probabilities. Similarly, the range of useful probabilities of either kind must not be constrained. These modifications allow a wider use from the earlier model "hypothesis-deductive (H-D)" to "hypotheses-inferential (H-I)." Keep in mind that Hempel's work on understanding explanation and prediction in science also applies to the branch of science in medical diagnosis (see chapters 5 and 6).

"Evidence-based medicine" (EBM) was launched in 1991 by G. Guyatt, Professor of Epidemiology at McMaster University in

Hamilton, Canada. This model of medical diagnosis differs sharply from traditional "H-I" (or earlier "H-D") models. To my knowledge, the EBM model continues to rule out medical theory and mechanisms, whereas traditional clinicians are prone to use their full medical knowledge in diagnosis. Up to date medical literature should be available to all clinicians in this country, along with its faults (e.g., not fresh, higher cost, and less accurate than the experienced clinician, especially for the patient with complex diseases). Such complexities demand analytic reasoning with theory and mechanisms (see chapters 8 and 9).

Statistical approaches may improve medical diagnosis by finding new correlations between empiric features among subjects. Typically subjects in clinical trials have been carefully selected for certain similarities and avoiding others (a protocol), hoping to minimize outliers. These are problematic. Some may be caused by mistake. On the other hand, an outlier may occur by an unknown causal feature like a tendency law (chapter 4). While this may be investigated and of scientific value, it brings us to a related topic: the individual patient.

Why is an unmistaken outlier different from all the non-outliers among the original subjects? Given no mistake, the answer should be clear: she/he has a feature different from others in the group, while everyone else in the group has differences from all others as well. Even identical twins are different at birth, with new differences in life history. Non-siblings have less genetics in common and in time more differences. Persons with sickness encounter new differences. Every person is human and is different in many ways—that is, unique. It can be difficult to see the individual patient from a bird's eye view.

CHAPTER 1

Kinds

At this time and places, most observers accept that medicine is a science, along with a kind of art in the patient-physician relationship. It is true that clinicians work in many different ways, a large proportion applying their scientific knowledge and methods in patient care, while other clinicians work at least partly in medical research and education. Clinicians who engage in research commonly involve human subjects, following protocols they or other clinicians have developed, and which are approved by Institutional Review Boards (IRBs). A majority of clinical researchers also spend a good portion of their time caring for patients. It is the science of medicine, involving both physicians and patients, that leads to new discoveries and deeper understanding of the human organism. Remarkably, human beings themselves, clinicians bring their minds, hearts, and hands to every aspect of the physician–patient encounters. These aspects can be seen as "kinds" in the science and art of medicine. The following list is of interest for our purposes, but is far from inclusive.

Diseases

According to D. Stanley and Campos, The International Classification of Diseases, 9th Revision (ICD-9) has 6,969 disease codes, and there are 12,420 codes in ICD-10 (WHO 2013).[3] These codes are designed to identify each known and classified disease, likely involving other diagnostic terms ("disorder," "condition," etc.). Surgical procedures are covered by other codes. These figures illustrate the extensive diversity of human disease and other maladies.

Symptoms and Signs

Conventionally, a "symptom" refers to a complaint by the patient. Examples are well known: pain, weakness, dizziness, etc. These complaints are subjective and not objectively measurable. Instead, a patient can often provide a subjective measurement, such as a number from an arbitrary scale (e.g., 1 – 10) of intensity of the complaint. This can usually be interpreted for significance by an experienced clinician.

A "sign" is an objective condition that can be normal or abnormal. Examples would include skin lesions, heart murmurs, etc. Unlike symptoms, signs can be to some extent objectively characterized by the clinician. Like symptoms, signs also can be graded for seriousness. Again, an experienced clinician will take note of significant abnormalities in her/his history and examination of the patient.

Note that a "sign" may itself count as a diagnosis, for example a bruise, mole, or laceration. Similarly, repeating clusters of certain signs and symptoms in various patients, lacking pathological understanding, may be diagnosed as a "syndrome." Over time, medical research may discover the explanatory pathophysiology of the syndrome, sometimes breaking it down into one or more "disease(s)," with new knowledge making these more amenable to treatment.

Causes and Correlations

Causes

Everyone (or nearly so) must be aware of the importance of causal relations in explanation of natural (macro) phenomena. This understanding is embedded in common knowledge and permeates our everyday decisions. Medical knowledge, research, and decision-making are similarly founded and supported by causal reasoning, both in creating new knowledge and everyday clinical applications.[4-7] Briefly put, a disease is the cause of its effects on the patient and the target of diagnosis.

Correlations

"Correlation" in a general sense indicates a connection or association between two or more entities. Such a connection may at times suggest a causal relationship. Here, temporal events are important. For example, suppose events A and B are correlated. If either event antecedes the other, it might be deemed causal in relation to the latter event, etc. Unfortunately, temporal events are often obscure, and pinpointing their advent not accurate. Sometimes, of course, a correlation can strengthen (or weaken) a causal relationship, especially in the context of a relevant theory. Otherwise, correlations can be difficult to interpret, whether relationships are like siblings (sharing causal antecedents), cousins, etc., or have no causal relations at all.

Logic: Deduction and Induction

These two kinds of argument are dominant in philosophy, especially in philosophy of science, and in scientific methods in general. They are very different.

Deduction

In every deductive argument, if its premises are true, its conclusion must also be true. The truth of the conclusion is guaranteed by the truth of the premises. There are many examples of this form of argument, such as:

All Studebaker cars are older than forty years.
This car is a Studebaker.

....

Therefore, this car is older than forty years.
Or:
All swans are white.
This bird is a swan.

....

Therefore, this bird is white

Both of these examples are logically correct. It is now known, however, that at least one species of swans are black, falsifying the general premise in the second argument. Falsification of natural "laws" in this manner has proved important in scientific methods.[8]

Induction

Inductive logic rests on the assumption that the future will be like the past—more precisely, that natural laws will hold in the future as in the past. This does not mean that if today's trajectory of climate warming should indeed despoil our planet that induction may have broken down (future unlike the past). On the contrary, both kinds of logic in science are warning us of such possible serious changes.

The premise supporting induction—that the future will be like the past—probably had doubters much earlier, but met its most serious challenges by David Hume. Hume, an eighteenth century Scottish philosopher (1711-1776), remains famous for his writings on the "problem of induction," with statements like, "How do you know that the future will be like the past?"[9]

Hume's question of induction is also an obstacle to cause and effect reasoning. I believe the best solution to this was developed by Karl Popper, a British philosopher from the mid-twentieth century. In the waning era of logical positivism and its claim that only confirmable empiric statements (including general laws) are meaningful, and other statements are metaphysical and without meaning, Popper proposed a new criterion for science: that its laws, theories, and hypotheses need only to be falsifiable. It turns out, as will be discussed later, that falsifying hypotheses is an inherent part of the diagnostic process.

Theory

A few days ago, I was amazed to read that physicists at the Gravitational-Wave Laboratory (LIGO) recently discovered a signal ("chirp") from detectors buried in tunnels. The detectors were designed to detect the effect of gravitational waves ("ripples") in space-time, emanating from a collision of two massive black holes. This collision occurred more than a billion light-years away from earth. The sensitivity of this experiment, and its results, are astonishing. It is also amazing that this new experimental result was predicted by Einstein's general theory of relativity about a century ago. Lawrence M. Krauss, the author of this article, states, "Science, like art, music, and literature, has the capacity to amaze and excite, dazzle and bewilder. I would argue that it is that aspect of science—its cultural contribution, its humanity—this is perhaps its most important feature."[10]

In common usage, the term "theory" has some semantic latitude. In physics and chemistry, for example, it would conventionally refer to higher-order generalizations of natural phenomena, sufficiently powerful to "explain" one or more lower–order empiric generalizations. Similar examples in medical science would include the germ theory in infectious diseases, feedback loops in homeostasis, immunology, genes, and so on.

Controversial in their origins, working theories are at times taken for granted but remain vulnerable to modification or replacement by new discoveries. Also in common usage, an uncertain empiric generalization—a simple hypothesis—may be viewed as theory. This could include something like "All swans are white," a statement that could not be proved, and in fact has been falsified. Many such generalizations are known to be only probabilistic, but nonetheless useful. This will be explored in later chapters.

Like all entities, we as human beings are subject to the laws of physics and chemistry, among others. And, like other sciences, medical science shares knowledge with many other sciences. In a few recent decades, physics and chemistry have been particularly useful in rapid advancements in medical imaging (e.g., CT, ultrasound, MRI, PET). "PET" (positron emission tomography, aka "molecular imaging") was developed in nuclear medicine, where injection or inhalation of radioactive agents allows special cameras to capture pictures of the "tracer" in the body. There are many types of tracer agents and uses. A tumor may accumulate an abnormal amount of the tracer, and be seen on a still image. After a heart attack (infarction), an abnormal amount of tracer accumulation at this site (still image), or may show an abnormal movement of a heart wall (video images).

Having worked in nuclear medicine in a good part of my career, and an early advocate for clinical use of PET (now established), a sketch of how this modality works might be an interesting example.

Several positron (same as an electron, but with a positive charge; aka "anti-matter") isotopes have been used in PET imaging (^{18}F, ^{13}N, ^{82}Rb, ^{11}C, ^{15}O ...). So far, ^{18}F has been the leader, having the best half-life (109.7 minutes) for most clinical purposes.

Remember that an emitted positron exists only until encountering an electron, when both particles mutually annihilate, spending their mass into two photons (energy), which move out in almost exactly opposite directions. If both photons are captured in suitably placed opposing detectors, with very accurate temporal windows (improved with "time-of-flight calculations),[11] their trajectories create an unseen line passing through the sphere of origin. I say "sphere," not "point," because the point of origin cannot be determined within the maximum annihilation range of the emitted positron. Fortunately, this decreases with a lower energy of the positron, and ^{18}FDG (a "labelled" molecule) has this advantage.

This is one more factor to consider: One line through a volume, e.g. a human chest or abdomen, would not be very satisfactory. However, a million, or several million, lines crisscrossing a sphere (or spheres) of origin in such a space, aided by a computer programmed for tomography, can be very effective in identifying lesions. In the case of [18]FDG, such lesions will typically be identified by their location and metabolic rate.

An analog of glucose, [18]FDG (^{18}F-flurodeoxyglucose) enters cells aided by glucose transporters. Unlike glucose, however, [18]FDG does not undergo glycolysis (metabolic breakdown) within the cell, raising its concentration. Its physical and chemical attributes has made [18]FDG a proverbial work horse in PET imaging, particularly in oncology. PET is used in other studies, however, some with different positron emitters and molecular carriers as well.

Finally, a word on the role of the physicians who determine when patients need this procedure, which parts of the body should be studied, appraisal of image quality (satisfactory?), interpretation of images, correlation of findings with images available from the past, and other imaging modalities (CT, MRI, ultrasound), whether which and when follow-up imaging is recommended. In cases involving investigative aspects, a specific protocol may add complexity. The physician leads a group of administrators, pharmacists, technicians, nurses, etc. She/he functions as a kind of maestro, directing trained and experienced players and is guided by their first priority: the best interest of the patient. Some may see this as a setting involving both science and art.

Keep in mind that observable phenomena and theory are not clearly separable. Rather, they merge into each other. Theories often use analogies taken from observable entities to frame models for theoretical entities. A classic example comes from work of the Danish physicist Niels Bohr early in the twentieth century, modelling the theoretic structure of the atom as analogous to the solar system. On the opposite side, there are many variants of what is observable, starting with pens and pencils, tables and chairs. In medicine, lacerations of the skin should be observable (if not too tiny, not covered, etc.).

For the surgeon removing a tumor in the lung of a patient, the tumor should be observable to her/him. Surely, the situation would be different for a physician looking for a similar tumor on a patient's lung by way of a conventional radiograph, due to assumptions and theory. The latter are greater by way of complex imaging, e.g., PET. In fact, even simple observables are not beyond mistake (an observer might have faulty eyeglasses, etc.). This will come up again.

Probabilities

This is a potentially large topic, partly because of its beginnings and of continuing interest in games of chance, and partly because of controversial perspectives on this subject. For present purposes, a general view of two major principles, and a little more, will suffice for needed purposes. Further discussion will come up in later chapters.

The Objective Perspective

Some philosophers and scientists prefer the mathematical approach to numeric chances of empiric events. This model has had many advocates, including R. A. Fisher, J. Neyman, K. Pearson, and E. Pearson, among others. They are the founders of much of modern statistical theory. Despite their advances (e.g., convergence theory), however, these theories have not overcome the problem of induction. Will the future be like the past, or how long is a sufficient "long run"? Nonetheless, this perspective has pragmatic uses.

The Subjective Perspective

A second general perspective on probability is called "subjective" or "belief" type. A belief type probability may be formed by personal experience and/or personal evidence. However, it is personally subjective. An important equation developed by Thomas Bayes (1702–1761), an English theologian, conforms well to use of this type. The "Bayesian" model will be further discussed in later sections.

A Thought Experiment

Imagine two farmers working in an ancient land. Curious and intelligent, they came upon a peculiar object, extremely similar to a modern die. It seemed to be solid stone, but with six equal square sides. For amusement, they colored the object, but curiously different on each side. They did not roll it. Knowing how to play games, one man offered to bet a coin if he rolled the object, hoping a specific color would come up. If willing to bet, how many coins should the second man bet against the given color? If a number were to enter her/his (or your) mind, how was it calculated? Was the object thought to be fair? Given only the description above, any probability calculation would be subjective—once known as a classic perspective. Based on common knowledge and human intelligence, it conforms neither to objective nor usual Bayesian probability theories.

A Second Thought Experiment

Sometime later, the same two characters described above stumbled upon something more exotic, e.g., a radio (perhaps left behind by an advanced alien space craft). They examined it, but of course the radio would not work (lucky for them!). They began to speculate and make bets on its origin and purpose. Having no previous experience with such an item, how accurate would be their speculations and bets? It's your guess. The point is that subjective probabilities really do have limitations.

Where to stand on probabilities?

We and our surroundings are continually subject to countless uncertainties, making necessary our use of probability in understanding (explaining) the past, and projecting (predicting) the future. Unswerving advocates (dogmatists) of probability theories exist on both sides of the objective and subjective divide. Some philosophers argue that we lean to both perspectives, as which best performs.[12] In general, some kind of middle of the road should be fitting, depending on the setting. Gamblers might prefer the objective route. In my view, physicians lean decidedly to the subjective perspective (not merely Bayesian) in diagnostic reasoning, calling on their knowledge and experience. However, both objective and subjective views have their uses and limitations.

REFERENCES AND FOOTNOTES:
INTRODUCTION AND CHAPTER 1

1. Groopman, J. "How Doctors Think," (2007) Houghton Mifflin Harcourt Publishing Company, New York, NY, p.24

2. Kirch W. and Schafil C., Medicine Vol 75, No.1 (1996) "Misdiagnosis at a University Hospital in 4 Medical Eras - Report on 400 Cases" pp29-40 In a study of 400 autopsy cases in a University Hospital (Germany), these investigators reported similar rates of ante-mortem misdiagnoses over a period of four decades. False positive rates were 7%, 11%, 9%, and 11%, respectively, whereas false negative rates were 24%, 39%, 29%, and 34%, respectively. These findings are similar to other earlier reports. Nonetheless, these authors conclude: "The introduction of new diagnostic procedures such as ultrasound, computerized tomography, and radionuclide scans has not reduced the rate of misdiagnoses. Misinterpretation, technical errors, and overreliance on these new procedures occasionally contributed directly to diagnostic errors. By contrast, the patient's medical history and physical examination played an important role in the diagnostic process, leading to a correct diagnosis in 60%–70% of cases." It should be noted that a decreasing rate of autopsies, performed more often in challenging cases, may bias such results against the rate of correct ante-mortem diagnoses.

3. Stanley, D, Campos, D, "The Logic of Medical Diagnosis" Perspectives in Biology and Medicine, (2013) vol.56 Num 2 (2013), pp300-315 The Johns Hopkins Univ. Press. Later a hospital staff reviewed ICD-10 (2018) and found total worldwide medical diagnoses of about 70,000.

4. Joyce, J. Phil. Stud. (2010) 147:139-154 "Causal Reasoning and Backtracking."

5. Okasha S. Oxford University Press (2002) "Explanation in Science" pp40-57
6. Hoerl C. Phil. Stud. (2011) 152 167-179 "Causal Reasoning"
7. Kwadsteniet L. J. of Evaluation in Clinical Practice, 19(2013) pp 112-117 "How do Practicing Clinicians Apply Learned Causal Information about Mental Disorders."
8. Rosenberg A., Philosophy of Science (2005), Routledge, New York, NY
9. Hacking I. "An Introduction to Probability and Inductive Logic," Cambridge University Press (2001), pp1-291
10. Lawrence M. Krauss, The New York Times, February 14, 2016.
11. Karp, JS et al, J Nucl Med, (2008), Mar49(3), "Benefit of time-of-flight in PET: experimental and clinical results." pp462-70
12. Hacking writes "We use one word, 'probability,' from both frequency and a belief perspective. That is no accident. We switch back and forth between the two perspectives." Hacking, I., "An Introduction to Probability and Inductive Logic," Cambridge University Press (2001), p 136

CHAPTER 2

Various Views of the Diagnostic Process

Introduction

Medical diagnoses, as claimed above, are not in general obvious to the clinician. Rather, they are typically the result of a more or less complex pattern of actions, observations, and reasoning on the clinician's part. A representation of a wider logical structure of this activity, the diagnostic process, will be developed in later sections. In this chapter, various other viewpoints and models about the diagnostic process will be explored.

The Statistical Interpretation

What can be described as a "statistical interpretation "[1] is a popular view of medical diagnosis among contemporary authors on the subject. One reason for this is the interest in adapting computer programs to aid medical diagnosis.[2-8] Another reason may be the many statistical generalizations in medical science and the admittedly probabilistic nature of much medical decision-making. A pioneer in this work, L. Lusted, in developing a statistical model of diagnosis, cites Osler: "Medicine is a science of uncertainty and an art of probability," and Pickering: "Diagnosis is a matter of probability, as those of us who follow the fate of our patients to post-mortem rooms know only too well. Prognosis is a matter of probability and in judging treatment we have to base our judgment on knowledge of probability."[9] However, general agreement in the spirit of these remarks need not include broad acceptance of the statistical model in diagnostic reasoning. Admitting the importance of statistical analyses and techniques in various facets of medical science, including aspects of diagnosis, it will be argued that the statistical formulations presented in medical literature have major shortcomings as diagnostic models for practicing physicians. I believe these shortcomings are sufficiently general to make unnecessary for our purposes detailed comparisons of various possible statistical approaches and their relative merits. Two such approaches will be discussed.

The Bayesian Model

Probably the most important statistical model of diagnosis, developed by several authors, especially Lusted,[9] is derived from Bayes' Theorem. The version commonly adopted for this purpose can be written as follows:

(1) $P(D/S) = P(S/D \cdot P(D)$

$$\overline{}$$

$$P(S)$$

where "D" is the proposition "disease D is present," "S" is the proposition "symptom (S) is present," etc. Expression (1) may then be read: the probability of the disease "D" given the symptom (or sign/symptom complex) "S" is equal to the probability of "S" given "D", multiplied by the ratio of the <u>prior probabilities</u> of "D" and "S". It is assumed (given the definition of "probability" utilized) that this equation is applicable to individual cases. Consider, for example, the case of a patient whose only known manifestations of illness are fever and painful throat of acute onset. Given this evidence, "S_j" (of course a clinician would want additional information before making a diagnosis), what is the probability in this patient of the disease "streptococcal pharyngitis," "D_s"? Using the above equation, the answer corresponds to the term "$P(D_s/S_j)$" and is equated with the term "$P(S_j/D_s)$" multiplied by the ratio "$P(D_s)/P(S_j)$." It may then be asked how these latter terms are defined and their values determined. Problems in the answer to this question raise the first of the following criticisms of this model.

Problem One: Statistics

The most common interpretation of these terms is their identification with incidence ratios. Hence, "$P(S_j/D_s)$" is identified with the incidence of the symptom-complex "S_j" among patients with the disease "D_s", and "$P(D_s)$" and "$P(S_j)$" respectively with the (statistical/

estimated) incidence of the given disease and of the symptom-complex in the population.

A problem with this interpretation is that incidence data are rarely known with the degree of reliability needed in this model, making such an approach generally impracticable. The difficulty is increased because if this term is defined by reference to "symptom-complexes" for given diseases, it will be considerably influenced by such things as the stage of the disease at the time of diagnosis, environmental factors including previous treatment, etc. (e.g., the effects of changes in dietary iodine intake on the prevalence and forms of thyroid disease). Hence, for this approach to be potentially useful, "P(S/D)" must be known for various populations and projected to an individual case from an appropriate specified population. The statistical information this would require is not generally available.

The situation in relation to the prior probabilities, "P(D)" and P(S)", is no better and may be worse. The incidence of a disease in a given population is rarely known with accuracy. This is likely to be more complex for a symptom-complex. The problem is compounded by the several-fold geographical and temporal variations in incidence of most diseases (e.g., as in streptococcal pharyngitis) and in symptom-complexes. While clinicians have some knowledge of these incidences, it is rarely more than broadly qualitative ("there is a lot of flu going around," etc.). Although this is commonly glossed over by proponents of the statistical model, it is not of minor importance.

Recognizing the deficiencies in the availability of incidence data, it is sometimes suggested that the values assigned to the above terms are derived from individual clinical experience and judgement. Given the clinician's knowledge, while the latter part of this suggestion is important, its soundness and scope does not derive from Bayes' Theorem, nor vice versa.

Problem Two: New Disease and Ideas

If medical diagnosis were confined to uses of the Bayesian model, there would be a difficulty in the introduction of new diagnostic concepts (designating new disease states). This is so if "P(D)" is taken as referring to incidence data. For whatever the real incidence of a disease, incidence data must relate to what has been observed, and in the case of a previously unrecognized disease the value for "P(D)" (and therefore "P(D/S)" must remain at 0. Moreover, this notion raises a false divide between clinicians and investigators, a flawed concept. This is clearly unacceptable. For centuries, physicians have shared new knowledge with others, including other sciences, in the care of patients. For example, Andreas Vesalius (1514-1564) and William Harvey (1578-1657), both physicians and investigators, described the human circulatory system, correcting earlier mistakes back to Hippocrates (460 -- 370 BCE), and Galen (130-216 CE).[10,11] One of the most important discoveries in all of medical science is the germ theory. Going back to the 10-11th centuries (Ibn Sina) and 15-16th centuries (Fracastoro), this theory came into bloom and practice in the nineteenth and early twentieth centuries. Mainstream scientists in this development included Louis Pasteur, a French chemist (1822-1895), and Joseph Lister, a Scottish surgeon (1827 – 1912). More recently and in this vein two Australian physicians made another major discovery, a bacterial cause for the majority of stomach and upper intestinal (peptic) ulcers. Their names are Barry Marshall (b.1951) and J. Robin Warren (b.1937). Dr. Warren, a pathologist, noted microscopic bacteria surrounding ulcers in patient specimens and showed them to Dr. Marshall, an internist. Together they worked for months to succeed with cultures of this newly discovered bacterium. Experimental trials in attempts to infect animals failed. Finally, Dr. Marshall decided to try infecting himself, drinking a potion of meat broth containing approximately one billion bacteria. Within a week he became quite ill (vomiting) and soon after underwent endoscopy, showing gastric inflammation and his stomach "swarming with bacteria."[12-14] Further experimenting by these physicians, and subsequently others, has shown that this infection can be cured. Named "Helicobacter Pylori," Dr. Marshall reports that this bacterium infects about half of the world's human population. Dr. Marshall and Dr. Warren received Nobel Prizes in 2005 for their work.

It may be said that while the importance of the physician's personal experience in regard to his decision making should not be ignored, and neither should it be overestimated, for the physician continually relates his own experience and reasoning to the framework of inter-subjective accepted theory and fact. The physician who works with patients having chronic pulmonary disease understands normal respiratory function in (about) the same way as other physicians, however seldom he encounters it among his patients.

There is a close relationship between the diagnostic process and the introduction of new, or the modification of old, diagnostic concepts, which the statistical model fails completely to illuminate, or to accommodate without physician meddling.

Problem Three: Faulty Probabilities

For diagnosis involving multiple signs and symptoms (the usual case), the Bayesian expression is accurate in a mathematically simple (multiplicative) way only if the phenomena described by relevant evidential statements—included in "S"—are statistically independent. This condition is often unmet. As one would expect, common manifestations of a given disease are as a rule not all independent.

A suggested approach in dealing with this problem would involve use of the general expression for Bayes' Theorem, written (Lusted):[15]

(2) $P(D/S_n, S_{n-1}, \ldots S_1) = P(S_n/D, S_{n-1}, \ldots S_1) \times P(D/S_{n-1}, \ldots S_1)$

$$\frac{}{P(S_n/S_{n-1}, \ldots S_1)}$$

Unfortunately, use of this expression would require statistical information far in excess of what is generally available. Lusted writes, "It is indeed difficult to imagine how, e.g., $P(S_n/S_{n-1}, \ldots S_1)$ could be practically determined."[16,17] Recognizing this, and calling what is needed "conditional independence," Lusted muses on potential ways around this problem. For example: "However, it may be possible to find some disease partition for which [symptoms] may well be conditionally independent ... If we are fortunate enough to define a group of diseases for which conditional independence for all symptoms and symptom complexes, then and only then may Bayes' theorem be written in the simple form of {(1)}."[18] While a solution this radical suggests the importance of the problem, this approach would seem for reasons having largely to do with the theoretic status of disease concepts a completely unacceptable basis for the definition, or attempted re-definition, of diseases.

This proposal, however, illustrates Lusted's sparse recognition of the causal connections between diseases and their clinical manifestations, a natural propensity among Bayesian advocates.

Another possible approach in eliminating the undesirable redundancy between co-dependent evidential variables would be the combination of these into (independent) clusters. Lusted suggests, "a thorough search throughout the entire medical field for groups or clusters of symptoms should result in a condensation of symptoms into clusters which would be easier to manage..."[19] Such a search or result has quite definitely not been accomplished, nor it seems has it been widely attempted. Feinstein, another pioneer and advocate in this movement, admits: "Existing survey data often list the total number of individual clinical properties present in a population, but seldom cite the co-existence and inter-relationship of *combinations of properties*."[20] (italics original)

A similar radical approach involves the exclusion of co-dependent kinds of evidence. For example, in a study of computer diagnosis of Cushing's Syndrome using a form of Bayes' Theorem, Nugent excluded for this reason "ecchymosis" and "low serum potassium" from the list of admissible data.[21] While one may preserve the formal correctness of the statistical model, attempts to eliminate the effects of redundancy between inter-dependent items of evidence, as by the routine exclusion of various kinds of evidence from relevance, do not accord well with the methods of ordinary clinical reasoning. Co-variance between manifestations of disease is context dependent. It will frequently vary with the stage of a given disease (e.g., serum enzyme changes in myocardial infarction), and it will vary between the diseases being considered. Similar manifestations of disease may in respect to one disease be variably dependent, and for other diseases not (or differently) so. The usual situation in differential diagnosis is, of course, consideration of diseases with similar manifestations. For example, the manifestations of low serum potassium and hypertension are (presumably) inter-dependent in Cushing's disease, but not so (or less so) in essential hypertension, although an iatrogenic correlation between them may in fact be found among patients with the latter diagnosis who have been treated with certain drugs.

Accordingly, the diagnostic usefulness of a certain disease manifestation is not always related to the degree of its independence. Co-dependent variables may be of decisive importance in many diagnostic contexts in spite of their apparent redundancy in relation to a given diagnosis from the statistical viewpoint, especially when the diagnosis is treated independently of competitors, as is often done in uses of the Bayesian model. For example, consider a simple situation in which "x" and "y" are common and co-variant manifestations of disease "A". Given that there may be several pathways to a certain manifestation, as is common, suppose disease "B" is also regularly accompanied by "x", but not by "y". The occurrence of "y", redundant in relation to "x" in the (Bayesian model) diagnosis of "A", will, however, be diagnostically uninformative about "A" (relatively) only in those contexts not requiring consideration of "B", which will in turn depend on consideration of other variables, etc. Moreover, co-variance of manifestations is rarely perfect, and while the occurrence of "y" in the presence of "x" may have little confirmatory value for "A" (in some contexts), its non-occurrence in such a situation may be strongly <u>disconfirmatory</u> for "A". Clinicians justifiably then continue to study and test the manifestations of disease in <u>detail</u>, omitting little or nothing of possible relevance, interpreting findings in their complex inter-relationships, including causal connections, in a manner appropriate to particular diagnostic challenges. From my perspective, these complex inter-relationships will not be easily or soon formalized.

Problem Four: Temporal Relations

Most presentations of the Bayesian model fail to account for the effects on diagnosis selection of different temporal relationships between manifestations of disease. Use of the cumbersome expression (2) would in practice be complicated by the fact that the values of its terms would in many cases be influenced by the temporal ordering of constituent items. In general, the probability of a manifestation "S_n" in a given disease with other manifestations "$S_1, ... S_{n-1}$" will depend on the order of appearance and duration of these manifestations. For example, in a patient habituated to the excess use of spirits, an abnormal glucose tolerance curve would be a probable finding given the manifestation(s) of recurrent bouts of pancreatitis, but the same could not be said of these manifestations in the reverse order. The probability of a disease in relation to a given set of manifestations will likewise vary with the order of their appearance, as in our example the probability of alcoholic pancreatic insufficiency as opposed to primary diabetes mellitus would vary. Modification of (2) to account for such effects would make its use even less practicable. The statistical model also fails to suggest or clarify the causal reasons for such effects.

Problem Five: Utilities

There are difficult problems in the formulation of diagnostic criteria, especially if based merely on statistically calculated probabilities. How probable must a disease be, or how much more probable than its possible competitors, to be accepted? How probable must a disease be, if dangerous to the patient, to justify further testing and/ or treatment, or if the disease could also be dangerous to others? I believe the manners in which clinicians deal with such problems have been grossly over-simplified or just neglected by many proponents of Bayesian (and other statistical) models for use in clinical diagnosis. There are scores of examples in the literature. Here's one that caught my eye: Discussing an attempt at such diagnosis, *based only on data from responses to a standard medical questionnaire*, an author writes, "In order to process a 'new' case, all that is required is the CMI [questionnaire]. For each disease, the sum of the significance values of the symptoms claimed is corrected for the patient's age and then divided by the mean age-corrected significance value for the disease. When this ratio, or likelihood index, reaches a predetermined minimum, the complex of symptoms claimed by the patient *identifies the patient as having the disease* (emphasis mine).[22] This is not acceptable. No matter where the predetermined minimum is set, and for obvious reasons it should not be set either too low or too high, I cannot imagine careful physicians being satisfied to diagnose or undertake treatment of a serious disease on such a basis. In the contemporary scene, it is true, many questionnaires are handed out to patients and being to some degree completed before seeing a physician. Fortunately, these questionnaires are used at best as a starting point for the physician, not an end point in the diagnostic process and treatment decisions.

The matter of diagnostic criteria is complex, in whichever way they are based. It is not always possible to formulate these for particular diseases[23] at all. Moreover, criteria for diagnosis, as well as for treatment, are viewed with vigorous skepticism by clinicians, who recognize the common deficiencies associated with their complexities and variability among individual patients. It is easy enough to add value or utility to calculated or estimated probabilities, by way of simple multiplication,[24] yet it is rarely done.[25] This goes to the crux of the matter: <u>Every patient is an individual case, and should be treated as one.</u> This is an important theme of this book, and it will be visited again.

Problem Six: The Role of Theory

What is perhaps the most important logical shortcoming of the Bayesian (or any other) statistical model of the clinical diagnostic process is that this model treats medical data as though it were neutral in respect to <u>theory</u>, whereas in general it is not. This is related to certain problems in the use of this model already discussed, e.g., in the modification of diagnostic concepts, the interpretation of variable dependency relations between manifestations of disease, and the importance of their temporal relations in diagnosis selection. Clinicians reason not only in terms of observed associations, but also by means of <u>causal</u> inferences based on accepted theory. There are ordinarily <u>theoretical</u> reasons guiding a clinician's inference from a hypothetical disease "A" to an expected manifestation "x". These reasons are related to her/his understanding of normal and abnormal processes in the human organism, and the various mechanisms (or "patho-physiology," etc.) of disease. The statistical model, embodying what might be called a black-box view of the organism,[26] fails completely to explicate the important relations between medical theory and clinical diagnosis.

Problem Seven: Dynamic Diagnosis

Disease is not like a still photograph but resembles a video continually evolving over time. Changes come about with the natural course of the disease, but also for other reasons, including treatment, sometimes based on a preliminary diagnosis. If signs and symptoms suggest a minor disease, such as a common cold, empiric treatment may suffice, obviating further testing and expense (remember the saying, "Take these tablets and call me tomorrow." The clinician's request for a follow-up call or visit is good judgment, as both the early diagnosis and its treatment can easily be wrong. Further exams and testing may be needed to correct the diagnosis, and <u>every treatment of the patient is itself a diagnostic test.</u> This interaction between the patient and her/his clinician(s) is critically important to the patient's outcome, and it takes time and focus on the individual patient. These real-life measures and their nuances are not easily made conformable to Bayesian or other statistical diagnostic models.

Problem Eight: Five Decades
of Progress and Failure

Progress:

Two major kinds of work with Bayesian models in medical diagnosis will be discussed. The first is the attempt to reduce the effect of co-dependent elements of evidence introduced to more complicated Bayesian models. These attempts largely follow Lusted's proposal to exclude redundant evidence. Holding with only statistical evidence, almost none of these models attempt to incorporate causal connections or pathophysiologic mechanisms,[27] with relatively few exceptions.[28-30] Other authors have reported that the simple ("naïve") Bayesian model performs as well compared to the more sophisticated versions.[31,32] Note that the latter of these two articles reports on a clinical study of the Long QT Syndrome in children. The authors comment, "These results suggest that data mining of clinical data in conjunction with a Bayesian modeling approach can lead to a diagnostic system for prediction of LQTS in children."[33] This kind of summation, having to do with machine diagnosis, is quite typical. In fact, I don't recall a report of poor results or frank failure. Odd?

Denekamp and Peleg, in a sterling article,[34] listed and analyzed eight models for computer aided diagnosis in use at that time. Most of these systems (not all Bayesian) have some special features, or not. Only one system "explicitly represents temporal relationships between data items."[35] Again, only one system fully, and another partly, "consider the geographic location of the patient as a factor in the diagnostic process."[36] Prefacing these issues, the authors acknowledge of these systems that "the rate of usage in clinical practice is low."[37] How could such important factors be missed?

Failure:

The marvels of medicine brought forth in the last five decades are well known, especially in the realm of technology in diagnostic methods. Practically unknown fifty years ago, CT, ECHO, MR, and PET are now household words in many parts of our society. These imaging modalities allow physicians to "see" not only detailed tomographic (3-D) internal anatomy, but also chemical/molecular kinetics and dynamic organ physiology within the patient. There can be no doubt that these advances have saved lives and improved many more. There can also be no doubt that these advances have depended on computers and other technology developments in the past fifty years, but this cannot be said about models developed during this time for use in machine (computer) diagnosis *per se*. Advocated by few, most clinicians do not like or use computer model diagnostics. Despite my interest in the subject, I can recall only one other clinician speaking about the Bayesian model, and who was also able to write its formula. Like their predecessors, the majority of clinicians remain busy interviewing, examining, testing, thinking about, and caring for every individual patient. After all, it's their responsibility.

Likelihood Ratios

Another statistical approach in medical diagnosis makes use of likelihood ratios. Lusted illustrates such a ratio as follows:[38]

(3) $$LR = \frac{P(S/D_i)}{P(S/D_j)} \quad (i \neq j)$$

in which the two terms are probabilities. Developed and named by the statistician R.A. Fisher (1890-1962),[39] this ratio can be variously interpreted in accord with whether "D_i" and "D_j" designate classes of patients with or without a given disease, or with one of two different diseases, respectively. The former interpretation dominates most discussion of likelihood ratios, whereas the latter can be more useful in understanding differential diagnoses.

Starting with the first interpretation, expression (3) can be re-written:

(4) $LR = P(S_i/+D_i)/\ P(S_i/-D_i)$

where "S_i" can denote a symptom or sign, or a <u>test result</u>, while "$+D_i$" and "$-D_i$" denote the presence or absence of disease "D_i," respectively.

Several authors have proposed use of nomograms, based on Bayes' theorem, to calculate binary diagnostic test results. This was first shown by TJ Fagan in 1975,[40] and has been further developed, by CG Caraguel and R Vanderstichel,[41] and most recently by L Herich, W Lehmacher and M Hellmich.[42] The latter group have constructed a non-electronic ruler, able on logarithmic scales to mechanically determine likelihood ratios, given other results from Bayes' Theorem.

Turning to the second interpretation of (3), equation (4) can be re-formed to express the likelihoods of two competing disease hypotheses as follows:

(5) $LR = P(Si/+Di)/\ P(Si/+D_j)$

These likelihood ratios can be incorporated in a Bayesian expression combining probabilities of the two disease hypotheses:

$P(D_i/S) = P(S/D_i)\ .\ P(D_i\ )$

(6) _____

$$P(D_j/S) = P(S/D_j) \cdot P(D_j)$$

Expression (6) has some positive aspects compared to (1). It brings out the important role in differential diagnosis that this process ordinarily requires. It also eliminates the murky term "P(S)." Its major deficiencies, however, belong to its statistical nature, making it subject to all of the problems that surround the Bayesian model.

To summarize important elements in the above criticisms, the statistical model of diagnosis severely misrepresents, in opposite ways, the state of medical knowledge and the clinician's use of such knowledge in medical diagnosis. On the one hand, this model exaggerates the availability of, and the need for, statistical data. On the other hand, it virtually ignores the much larger body of available medical knowledge and the central role of theory and causal inference in the clinician's diagnostic reasoning.

Algorithms: Decision-Tree and Related Models

Recognizing the sequential nature of decisions in clinical diagnosis, this process is sometimes represented by means of decision trees, discrimination nets, or algorithms. Harking again back to Lusted,[43] his proposals may be presented in forms like the following:

A Discrimination-Net Model

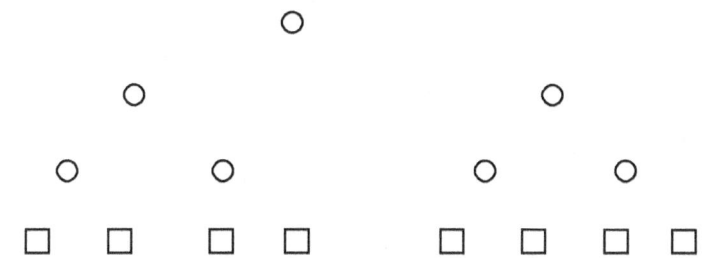

A Decision-Tree Model

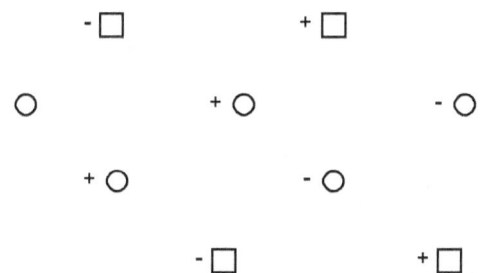

Each circle or square represents a specific question, and possible progression at each step is determined by whether the answer to the corresponding question is (+) or (-). The process continues until the clinician is satisfied with a diagnosis.

In this scheme, each circle corresponds to a specific question (or test) and equal square corresponds to a disease (or disease category). Whereas the decision tree model depicts a particular course of clinical inference, this model schematizes alternative inferential routes, each leading to a different diagnostic outcome. The discrimination net model may thus be seen as a conjunction of more than one decision tree, and importantly illustrates the usual situation in differential diagnosis, where evidence is evaluated in relation to several possible diagnoses.

Now generally called algorithms, these models have to some extent grown in familiarity, especially in programs aimed at computer aided diagnosis. However, their underlying concepts have been advanced primarily by psychologists. As I see it, and briefly, a prominent theme in the literature deals with a dual process theory, or "System 1 and System 2" diagnostic reasoning. System 1 deals with fast mental processing, whereas System 2 is slow, analytic, and reflective. These dual mental systems are widely accepted.[44] K. Stanovich has gone a bit further, proposing a tri-partite amendment to the theory, integrating both System 1 and System 2, but with System 2 more powerful, such that "Decoupling processes enable one to distance oneself from representations of the world so that they can be reflected upon and potentially improved."[45] Further refinements seem likely.

System 1 bathes in less glory, dealing with quick judgements, sometimes called "heuristics" (unfortunately).[46.47] Fast thinking may apply in a basic model of medical diagnosis known as pattern recognition. An example might be hyperthyroidism, an endocrine disorder with manifestations often easily recognized. However, this disorder can develop from several different causes. Most clinicians would thus not make a complete or proper diagnosis, sufficient for rendering treatment, without further information: questions, exams, and tests. Then even more information (including consultations) may be needed. Similarly, other observable disorders (skin lesions, fractures, etc.) commonly call for testing (biopsy, x-ray, etc.). Pattern recognition involving less observable evidence, such as test results, becomes more complex as medical science advances and expectations of accuracy increase. This is not to dismiss pattern recognition, which can play a significant role in the diagnostic process, to be discussed.

As for quick thinking, it first needs to be accurate and directed to the welfare of the patient, abilities gained from the scientific knowledge and experience of clinical medicine.[48]

Algorithmic models may be of some use in limited situations (e.g., if appropriate, computer-aided diagnosis). As accounts of the general diagnostic process, however, they are inadequate.[49] Their shortcomings include:

(a) They greatly oversimplify diagnostic decision-making. Clinicians deal not only with yes and no answers, but with all degrees of "maybe." Moreover, clinicians know how to deal with uncertainties, but these maneuvers are not clarified, or even indicated, by these models. The diagnostic process is far more complex than such models require.

(b) These models relate more to the psychology of the diagnostic process than its logic. The decision-tree model has in fact been developed by means of "think-aloud" studies of diagnostic problem-solving. As one would expect, it has been found that various clinicians use very different reasoning to arrive at a diagnosis. Lusted made this observation: "The number of branches in a particular decision-tree seems to be a function of the experience and ingenuity of the diagnostician. For the same diagnostic problem, one diagnostician may use a decision-tree with four branches whereas another diagnostician may use forty."[50] The algorithmic models provide no answer to the question how by such different routes, which may be long and complex, clinicians so often arrive at a common diagnosis.

(c) Once set to work, these models have a natural tendency to harden. To serve their purpose, of course, they must be endowed with some kind of esteem. As things are in our country, medical insurance and litigation play a role in these aspects. Doctor J. Groopman writes, "Algorithms discourage physicians from thinking independently and creatively. Instead of expanding a doctor's thinking, they can constrain it."[51] I will argue later that this is not the way to further the best interests of patients, physicians, and the science of medicine.

In summary, while algorithmic models may serve to illustrate some features of the diagnostic process, providing pictorial representations of possible roadmap approaches in certain contexts, they do not adequately explain the logic of clinical reasoning. A more general and satisfactory view of this process will be explored.

REFERENCES AND FOOTNOTES: CHAPTER 2

1. I use the term "statistical" for want of a better one. This aligns some-
    what with Hacking's notion quoted above (#12). In fact, Bayes' formu-
    lation works with numbers from either objective or subjective sources,
    or a mix. The word "mathematical" comes to mind, but numbers are
    not available in many subjective uses of Bayes' theorem. This poses a
    problem in such uses in medical diagnosis, as will be discussed.

2. Gil C. BMJ Vol. 337 (May 2005) "Why Clinicians are Natural
    Bayesians." pp1080-1083

3. Svolos P. et el, Clinical Imaging 37 (2013) "Classification methods for
    differentiation of atypical meningiomas using diffusion and perfusion
    and techniques at 3-T MRI." pp856-864

4. Liu Y. AJR 196:May (2011) "A Bayesian Network for Differentiating
    Benign from Malignant Thyroid Nodules Using Sonographic and
    Demographic Features" W598-W604

5. Qu L., et al IEEE International Conference on Bioinformatics and
    Biomedicine (2010) "A Naïve Bayes classifier for differential diagnosis
    of long QT syndrome in children" pp433-437

6. Herrle S. et al, Acad Med(2011) May 86(5) "Bayes Theorem and
    the Physical Examination; Probability Assessment and Diagnostic
    Decision-Making" pp618-627

7. Vab der Sus H. J ASM Med Inform Association (2006):13
    "Overriding of drug safety alerts in computerized physician order
    entry" pp 138-147

8. Ashutosh K Journal of Clinical and Diagnostic Research (2011)
    April Vol-5(2)"Differential diagnosis:" Cases with equal Posteriori
    Likelihoods." p418

9. Lusted L. "Introduction of Medical Decision-Making." Springfield
    Ill.: Charles C. Thomas, 1968

10. Nutton V. "Humours and Pneumas" in "Great Discoveries in Medicine" Editors Bynum W. & Bynum H., Thames and Hudson, London, Ltd. UK (2011) pp26-28

11. Ford J. "Circulation" in "Great Discoveries in Medicine" Edited by Bynum w. & Bynum H., Thames and Hudson, London Ltd UK (2011)" pp56-59

12. Marshall B. "Helicobacter Pylori & Peptic Ulcer" "Great Discoveries in Medicine" Edited Bynum Bynum W., & Bynum H., Op Cit. pp288-290

13. It is generally known that patients often participate in approved experimental medical studies. Many physicians and other medical staff do so also, particularly in academic centers.

14. Marshall B. Op Cit. p290

15. Lusted L. "Decision-Making Studies in Patient Management." New England Journal of Medicine." :416-424 February 1971 Note that on our interpretation of "S" as a proposition the appropriate connective here is "and," with "S" identical with "S1 & S2 ... Sn," etc.

16. Ibid, pp 416-424

17. Note that on our interpretation of "S" as a proposition the appropriate connective here is "and," with "S" = "S1 & S2 & ... Sn", etc.

18. Defined as holding when $P(S/D) = P(S1/D) P(S2/D)$, where "S" = "S1 & S2". Lusted, op cit. p 18

19. Lusted, ibid, pp 17-18

20. Feinstein, A.R. : Scientific Methodology in Clinical Medicine." Annals of Internal Medicine 61: 944-965. 1964. Italics original.

21. Nugent, C.A. "The Diagnosis of Cushing's Syndrome," in Jacquez, J.A. (ed.): The Diagnostic Process (Proceedings of a conference held at the University of Michigan, May 1963) Ann Arbor, Mich.: Malloy Litho., Inc., 1964

22. Goldstein, L. S. "Data Processing and the Interpretation of Symptoms," in Jacquez, op. cit. 242-243.

23. Zhang, W. et al, Annals of Rheum Dis. 2010: 69:"EULAR evidence-based recommendations for the diagnosis of knee osteoarthritis" pp483-489

24. Hacking I. Op cit p79

25. O'Connor P JAMA August 10, 2005 Vol 294 No 06, "Adding Value to Evidence-Based Clinical Guidelines." pp741-743

26. Lusted, l. Op cit. p 20

27. Denekamp, Y., and Peleg M., "TiMeDDx – A multiphase anchor-based diagnostic decision-support model." J. of biomedical informatics 43 (2010) pp 111-124

28. Peng Y. et al, AAAI-Proceedings (1986) (www.aaai.org) +Plausibility of Diagnostic Hypotheses: The Nature of Simplicity" pp 140-144

29. Console L et al, IJCAI'89 Proceedings of the 11th international joint conference on Artificial Intelligence – Volume 2 (Automated Reasoning Techniques for Intelligent Systems) and CNR of Italy, Torino, Italy, "A Theory of Diagnosis for Incomplete Causal Models" pp 1311-1317

30. Lucas P. Artificial Intelligence in Medicine 5 (1993) Elsevier "The representation of medical reasoning models in resolution-based theorem-provers" pp 395-414

31. Domingos P. Machine Learning, 29 (1997) Kluwer Academic Publisher, The Netherlands "On the Optimality of the Simple Bayesian Classifier Under Zero-One Loss," pp 103-130

32. Qu L. IEEE International Conference on Bioinformatics and Biomedicine (2010) "A Naïve Bayes Classifier for Differential Diagnosis of Long QT Syndrome in Children" pp 433-437

33. Qu L., ibid., p 433

34. Denekamp Y. and Peleg M., op cit., P 114

35. ibid., p.114

36. ibid., p. 114

37. ibid., p.111

38. Lusted, L. (1968) op cit., p 20.

39. Hacking, I. (2001) Op cit., p.225 Note that Hacking finds the term "likelihood ratio" confusing, as it sometimes functions like "probability," but not always. One possible confusing factor is that likelihood ratios become additive only when in logarithmic form, unlike probabilities.

40. Fagan TJ N Engl J Med 1975;293 Letter: "Nomogram for Bayes theorem." p.257

41. Caraguel CG, and Vanderstichel R, Evid Based Med 2013;18 "The two-step Fagan's nomogram: ad hoc interpretation of a diagnostic test result without calculation." pp125-128

42. Herich, L., Lehmacher W., and Hellmich M., Methods of Informatic Medicine, January 2015 "Drop the Likelihood Ratio: A Novel Non-electronic Tool for Interpreting Diagnostic Test Results" pp1-5

43. Lusted, L., Op cit., pp 74-75

44. Croskerry P. Academy Medicine, vol 84, number 8/August 2009 "A universal model of diagnostic reasoning." pp 1022-1028

45. Stanovich K. Oxford University Press. In Evans J.,"In two minds: dual processes and beyond," "Distinguishing the reflective algorithmic and autonomous minds: is it time for a tri-partite theory?" pp55-80

46. The term "heuristic" here defined as a "short cut" is confusing, as the term has also meant teaching to stimulate investigation or discovery, a nicer definition. What's wrong with calling a short cut a "short cut?"

47. Pople, H E. In Szolovits (Ed) "Artificial Intelligence in Medicine" Westview Press. Boulder, Colorado 1982 "Heuristic methods for imposing structure on ill-structured problems: the structuring of medical diagnostics." pp2-57.

48. Groopman, J., Op cit., pp5-6, 238-239

49. Groopman, J. Op cit. pp 5-6

50. Groopman J Op cit. p6

51. Groopman, ibid., p6

CHAPTER 3

Covering Law and Hypotheses–Inferential Model

Introduction

What may be called "the covering-law hypotheses-inferential model" of clinical diagnosis has been with us for several decades. Relating the diagnostic process to a deductive model, these early authors note, "the clinician lists his possible diagnoses" and "tests each hypothetical diagnosis in turn, trying to disprove the incorrect and to prove the correct."[1] Furthermore, "he does this by asking two questions: Does the diagnosis explain the findings? And, are the expected findings present?"[2] Summarizing the brief but insightful discussion, these authors conclude, "Differential diagnosis, like scientific research, is ... based on the method of hypothesis."[3]

The ideas involved in this model of diagnosis are neither new nor novel. They were, for example, expressed several further decades ago by Cabot, who wrote of "forming reasonable hypotheses about a case of disease" and then "testing these hypotheses by such experiments as shall establish the correct and nullify the incorrect." That "each case should lead us to arrange before the mind's eye a selected group of reasonably probable causes for the symptoms complained of and for the signs discovered," and that "every item of physical or chemical examination is an experiment made to test the soundness of an idea about the case in hand."[4] Later discussing the "developing and testing of clinical hypotheses" in medical education, Engle writes, "the instructor points out how the process of clinical investigation, beginning from the moment the physician meets his patient, inevitably involves developing a series of hypotheses, which are successively tested in the course of the continuing interview and examination," and that "many different types of hypotheses may properly be entertained."[5] In a similar vein, Almy writes of a particular diagnosis that it "must be based upon (1) the recognition of characteristic symptoms, (2) the exclusion of other disease processes suggested by the symptoms and (3) repeated and conscientious testing of the hypothesis."[6]

Not surprisingly, some recent authors have supported this model, intermingling use of causal connections, statistical numbers, and subjective probabilities.[7-10] Essentially, all such articles have been putatively based on hypothesis-deductive reasoning. As discussed in chapter one, however, true deductive reasoning does not generally belong in arguments involving uncertainty (hence, the title "hypotheses-inferential" is used in this model).

What is surprising is that while often implicitly recognized, this model has received so little discussion in most modern writings on the diagnostic process, for it provides the best means for understanding the logic of this process. It has the following immediate apparent conceptual advantages:

(1)   It properly draws and emphasizes the commonly recog-
        nized distinction between a disease and its manifestations,
        and the fallacy of identifying the former with, or trying to
        deduce it from, the latter. This distinction, which permits
        development of the role of theory in the diagnostic process,
        is commonly glossed over in statistical accounts.

(2)   It properly emphasizes the importance of the list
        of differential diagnoses in respect to a given set of
        manifestations, and the traditionally important method of
        diagnosis by exclusion. On this account, the probability of
        a certain disease is enhanced not only by evidence that is
        confirmatory for that disease, but also by evidence that is
        disconfirmatory for other diseases, which would otherwise
        account for the same manifestations. The nature of the
        clinician's search for evidence, a process of critical testing
        dependent on his understanding of disease mechanisms
        (along with prevalence, co-morbidities, patient desires, etc.),
        and directed in relation to a set of differential diagnoses,
        is clarified.

(3)   This model asserts, as its designation suggests, that there are
        inferences involved in clinical diagnosis. Since diagnostic
        statements and statements about disease manifestations in a
        given case are ordinarily all singular propositions, and since
        in general a singular proposition cannot be inferred from
        another singular proposition (with certain exceptions),[11]
        this model demands an account of the role of scientific law-
        like statements in the diagnostic process. This requirement
        seems highly relevant and appropriate.

Other apparent merits of this model will be developed in later discussion. An understanding of the diagnostic process based on this model would, for example, support a methodological shift away from the present emphasis on confirmatory findings. Such an understanding would also have important, if less tangible, ramifications in relation to the clinician's scientific role, the objectives of medical education, various socio-legal aspects of medicine, etc. In pursuit of this understanding, the following sections will be devoted to an explication of the structure and uses of the hypotheses-inferential model in the light of a general account of the logic of scientific explanation.

Diagnostic Propositions: Their Structure and Functions

Structure

As was stated earlier, diagnostic propositions ("John Jones has measles") are ordinarily singular propositions. The subject term of a diagnostic proposition denotes an individual patient. The predicate term of such a proposition, which typically designates a disease, is more problematic and more interesting. The various ways in which these predicate terms are <u>defined</u> have a great deal to do with the logic of their use (i.e., with the confirmation of their corresponding diagnostic propositions, etc.). In this respect, recognizing that for other purposes different classifications may be used, three important classes of disease will be briefly examined based on their modes of <u>definition</u>.

(1)   <u>Diseases defined in terms of a single observable feature.</u>[12]

There are many possible examples of this, e.g., "alopecia" or "mole." Most of these, quite naturally, have to do with the exterior aspects of the organism. Many injuries (traumatic diseases) would also fall into this group, e.g., "laceration of the arm."

The logic regulating the use of diagnostic propositions such as these is apparently quite straightforward: they can be verified or disproved (ignoring possible observer <u>error</u>) by a simple act of observation. The matter may be complicated in fact by possible ambiguity or disagreement in the disease definition. Such disagreement may arise from (relatively unproblematic) differences in the restrictiveness with which the corresponding normal state is defined (e.g., "Is there sufficient redness present to be pharyngitis?") Disagreement may also arise from more problematic differences in the <u>interpretation</u> of the observed characteristic in relation to suspected disease etiology and pathogenesis (e.g., "Is this a furuncle or a carbuncle?"). For clinical observation, like observation elsewhere, it is not immune to the influence of theory.

There is a way in which theory has limited the practical importance of disease concepts as in category (1). For useful refinements in disease concepts, occurring with the development of medical science, have usually come about as a result of increasing reference in their definition to unobservable events or processes. Hence, while fever was at one time considered a disease, it is now quite uniformly regarded as only a manifestation of various diseases. Similarly, some clinicians would not now be content with the diagnosis of pharyngitis, but would seek its refinement in, for example, etiologic terms, as in streptococcal pharyngitis.[13]

Thus, while the class of diseases defined in the above manner may provide a model of the theory of manifest medical diagnoses, the model is certainly not generally applicable, for this manner of disease definition is of limited utility.

(2) <u>Diseases defined in terms of multiple observable features.</u>

In this class, consisting mainly of the traditional group of medical syndromes, the meaning of a diagnostic term "D" is derived entirely from the specification of a set of observable features, e.g., "$S_1, S_2 \ldots S_n$". In the ideal case, the formal principle regulating the use of the corresponding diagnostic term can be expressed as follows:

If, and only if, $(S_1, S_2, \ldots S_n)$, then D.

This is just a logical equivalence. The only inference involved in making such a diagnosis is the passage to (or from) the <u>definindum</u> from (or to) the <u>definiens</u>. Given the needed specification of features (including appropriate temporal as well as spatial reference), such a diagnostic proposition can, as in (I), be verified or disproved by any observer who has the requisite findings and understands the definition. A number of additional comments can be made on interesting features of this class of diseases.

(a) The simple regulatory principle (I) is rarely applicable in practice. For most syndromes, clinicians are not able to specify definitely the features $S_1, S_2, \ldots$, etc. It is often the case that while each member in a given set of features $S_1, \ldots S_n$ may be considered <u>relevant</u> to the diagnosis of a certain syndrome, these features are often not held to be <u>jointly necessary</u> for the diagnosis. Rather, various possible subsets of these features may be considered sufficient. Moreover, not only may the <u>necessary</u> characteristics "S_1, S_2, . . ." of a syndrome be difficult to specify, but questions may arise concerning their <u>sufficiency</u> as a diagnostic criterion. These may come about in various ways. For example, in addition to its defining characteristics, a syndrome will ordinarily have known associations with other (non-defining) manifestations, the absence of which would—at least in some cases—cast doubt on the correctness of the diagnosis. The same effect may result from the presence of other manifestations, not mentioned in its definition, either as these may be known to be causally more or less incompatible with the syndrome (e.g., hypoglycemia in relation to Cushing's syndrome), or as they may lie beyond that for which the correct diagnosis (remembering that <u>sometimes</u> a combination of diagnoses may be required) is held accountable. Features such as these are routinely uncovered in the process of diagnostic evaluation in individual cases, where a syndrome diagnosis, like others, must ordinarily undergo a <u>process of testing</u>, which may sometimes result in its rejection in favor of competing diagnostic possibilities.

Uncertainty concerning which combinations of features justify use of a given syndrome diagnosis is associated with a degree of vagueness in the corresponding diagnostic concept. Disease concepts defined in general conformity with (2) are in fact often quite inexact. Clinicians attempt to sharpen such concepts by thinking in terms of idealized or classic cases. It is

only in such cases, infrequently encountered, that the
formulation (I) would seem applicable.[14]

(b)   Clinicians are rarely if ever satisfied with a syndrome
concept of disease. There is a central assumption in clinical science that for syndromes there exist some (one or
more) etiologic event or process.[15] Their discovery, with
advances in medical science, usually results in modification of corresponding disease concepts, which have
thereby come increasingly to reflect causal relations and
distinctions. Many syndrome disease concepts have
been thus modified with clarification of their relevant
etiologic processes. This modification typically occurs
in the defining of a new set of diseases, in relation to
a given syndrome, in which causal factors and distinctions are appropriately accounted for. When this takes
place, features that function as defining characteristics
of the syndrome (disease?) come to be seen as mere
manifestations of one or more diseases. An example
of this is Cushing's syndrome, defined by reference to
certain features (most would agree observable), which
is now known to be a possible expression of a variety of
diseases of which the etiologically defined Cushing's
disease is but one. Similar considerations apply to an
opposite condition, like the Addison syndrome, etc.
Thus, while syndromes continue to be important in
medicine—regularities between the manifestations of
disease are important—they are regarded by clinicians
less as adequately defined diseases than as the effects of
other more or less well-defined disease(s).

(c)   The preceding discussion brings into focus the previously noted distinction between two aspects of a
disease, its cause and its manifestations. Both of these
aspects may play a part in the definition of a disease.
The relative weights of these parts is a complex and
variable matter. Much depends, of course, on how
much is known about the causal mechanisms involved.
In general, however, when the cause of a disease is
known it becomes an important criterion (setting
aside the matter of its detection) for the presence of
the disease, and assumes a corresponding importance
in defining the disease concept. It may be contended,
moreover, that it is not only true in fact but important
that disease concepts should embody causal distinctions, for it is by virtue of such distinctions that rational search for modes of treatment of different diseases
is possible.[16,17]

(d)   Finally, it should be pointed out that many of the causal
events in disease are not themselves observable—or
are observable only by special techniques—and are
often highly theoretical (e.g., genetic, biochemical, or
cellular abnormalities, etc.).[18] The role of theoretical
concepts in clinical diagnosis will be taken up in subsequent discussion. It should be clear, however, that the
method of diagnosis expressed in (2) will not hold for
any disease defined wholly or in part by reference to
unobservable entities or processes, in particular theory.
Inasmuch as such disease concepts are in fact common,
the diagnostic principle (1) must again be seen as not
generally applicable.

This conclusion might be circumvented only by extending the sense of syndrome (or (1)) beyond what has been indicated above to include such observables (e.g., laboratory measurements) as <u>refer to</u> appropriate theoretic, or otherwise unobservable phenomena. This maneuver, amounting to an operational re-definition of relevant theoretic terms, may be fitted for diagnosis by statistical or computer methods. It has the important disadvantage, though, of obscuring known and useful <u>causal</u> distinctions and relations between theoretic and manifest features of a disease. Inasmuch as these distinctions and relations are important in clinical reasoning, as they certainly are, such a maneuver would serve to muddle rather than to clarify medical diagnosis and should be rejected in a general account of this process.[19] These considerations lead to the following major class of diseases.

Diseases defined wholly or in part by means of theoretical terms.

Some intimations of what is meant by "theoretical" terms in this context have already been given. Certainly to be included in this group are <u>at least</u> those terms that refer to entities or processes that are unobservable by any available technique. Examples of medical diagnoses containing such terms are the presence of unusual amounts of various types of hemoglobin molecules in the red blood cells, diagnoses asserting various biochemical derangements, etc. Perhaps less obviously but also to be included are such pathophysiologic diagnoses as myocardial ischemia, which asserts a deficiency of oxygen (and other molecules) in the heart muscle relative to its functional requirements. Yet to be included are such diagnoses as viral hepatitis, a compound term including a relatively more theoretic term "virus" (observable, if at all, by means of electron microscopy, the interpretation of which depends on theory) and an apparently less theoretic term "hepatitis." The definition of even this latter term, however, involves theoretic components (e.g., interpreting what is seen through the light microscope, its involvement of theoretic concepts of inflammation, biochemical derangements, etc.).

There are many other examples of diagnostic predicates whose definitions are thus comprised of a blend of theoretic and observational terms. It is fair to say that the definitions of most diagnostic terms in modern medicine are of this kind, being more or less influenced by theory. It is moreover reasonable to expect this to become increasingly true with advances in understanding of disease mechanisms, as these link theoretic processes to disease manifestations. An example of this trend is the above-mentioned viral hepatitis, which is now a more acceptable diagnosis than "yellow jaundice." Consider again the disappearance of the diagnosis "fever." Another example is the shift in our concept of "diabetes mellitus." Diagnosed in antiquity by the quantity and sweetness of the urine (as the name implies), clinicians are now diagnosing chemical forms of the disease without clinically observable manifestations.[20] It may be worth quoting a medical definition of this disease, containing a blend of reference to theoretical and observable phenomena, and their complex causal relationships. Hence, a definition: "Diabetes mellitus is a group of metabolic diseases characterized by hyperglycemia resulting from defects in insulin secretion, insulin action, or both. The chronic hyperglycemia of diabetes is associated with long-term damage, dysfunction, and failure of various organs, especially the eyes, kidneys, nerves, heart, and blood vessels."[21] Interestingly, the "group of metabolic diseases" in this citation replaces the older classification of one disease with "Type 1 and Type 2," engrained in greater knowledge of pathogeneses in this spectrum of disease. This increased knowledge allows better treatment.

Diabetes mellitus is an example of a diagnostic term that has survived for centuries in spite of changes in both its definition and its empiric conditions of use, brought about by advances in medical science. However, such advances have sometimes (as with "ether" in physics) resulted in the virtually complete disappearance from clinical use of once important diagnostic terms (e.g., chlorosis).

The importance attributed to theory in the language of clinical medicine is reinforced by two further considerations. The first is that the influence of theory is evident not only in the definition of diseases, as discussed, but also in other clinical terms that function in putative observation reports. An example of this is the term "opening snap," which not only describes a certain kind of heart sounds, but also carries implicit reference to its etiology and pathogenesis. The theoretically interpretative (or "theory-laden") nature of such observation reports is a potential (and probably not uncommon) source of disagreement among clinicians in their use.[22]

Second, it has in recent times been argued that there is no pure observational language, i.e., that all intersubjective descriptive predicates, including observational terms, are to some extent theory-dependent in their meaning and use. Accepting the view that the distinction between observational and theoretical predicates is one of degree and not one of kind, i.e., that these terms are not separated by a logical gap, does not however mean that this distinction is not yet for some purposes useful or important. It is important, for example, in the separation of disease classes above.

Advocates of this view do not shun occasional use of the distinction. Moreover, some form of the distinction is necessary to an account of the differences between terms (and their uses) that refer respectively to highly observable (e.g., billiard balls) or certainly unobservable (e.g., neutrons) <u>entities</u>. Some disease predicates are defined at least in part by reference to such unobservable entities, and it seems useful to distinguish such relatively theoretic terms (and the logic of their use in diagnosis) from such clearly observational terms as "superficial laceration." While the latter term may be regarded as to minor degree theory dependent, and the stability of its definition and criteria of use may be ascribed to a high degree of theoretic entrenchment, it would nonetheless appear a mistake not to distinguish the usual manner of application of this term from that of such relatively theoretic terms as "Glucose-6-Phospho-Dehydrogenase Deficiency," or "myocardial calcium blocker," etc.

Accordingly, while the recognition that observational terms are to varying degrees theory-dependent provides an important insight, this insight should not be exaggerated to obscure, for example, such pragmatically important differences as there may be in the normal methods for use of these terms. However, the extent to which observational terms are more rather than less theory-dependent does not detract from but instead clearly supports the importance of medical theory in clinical diagnosis.

Finally, it is worth noting that the use of many diagnostic predicates that refer to entities or processes in a sense observable, but only by imaging procedures (or by the surgeon or pathologist), influencing the level of theory. Such entities (organs, tissues, fluids) and processes are for obvious reasons not always observable in the usual sense to the clinician in typical diagnostic settings.

Far from being a peripheral or subordinate matter, medical theory plays a central importance in clinical diagnosis, and an examination of this role to be of corresponding importance in understanding the diagnostic process. Analysis of this role will require discussion of the use of law-like statements and scientific inference in medical diagnosis. These topics will be taken up after a few comments on the uses of diagnostic propositions.

Functions

Major functions of diagnostic propositions in clinical use are two-fold. The first is:

A Descriptive Function

That diagnostic propositions <u>describe</u> is clear from what has already been said. They attribute some property or state (more or less theoretic) to an individual patient. Of course, not every statement fulfilling this condition is a diagnostic proposition. What distinguishes the diagnostic propositions of clinical medicine from other singular propositions about humans? No hard and fast line of demarcation is evident. Apart from convention, and the requirement of empiric content (they must be empirically testable), an important distinguishing feature of diagnostic propositions is that their predicate terms form an integral part of organized medical science. This feature is connected with the second major function.

An Explanatory Function

Diagnostic propositions function not only descriptively, ascribing to some patient a certain property or state (ordinarily a disease), but they serve in the explanation of other properties of the patient. Hence, we may say of Mr. Smith that he is weak because he has some type of anemia. Moreover, explanations involving diagnostic concepts frequently include several levels. Mr. Smith's anemia, for example, may itself be explained in relation to another disease (e.g., atrophic gastritis, ileitis, ulcer), as congestive heart failure may similarly be explained in relation to valvular heart disease, coronary artery disease, or thyrotoxicosis.

In addition to diagnostic propositions, such explanations clearly require the use of generalizations and law-like statements. In the case of Mr. Smith's weakness, e.g., concerning the functions of hemoglobin in oxygen transport and oxygen in metabolism, which are part of medical science and not simply whimsical or sporadic. This qualification, relating to the <u>use</u> of diagnostic propositions in medicine, further distinguishes these from other empiric statements. Thus, while the proposition "Mr. Jones is 7'2" tall" may express a fact of clinical importance for certain purposes (e.g., in respect to the diagnosis of various endocrine diseases), it is not a diagnostic proposition (it does not predicate anything resembling a disease), and it would serve few if any explanatory functions in medicine. An explanation involving its use, by way of contrast, of why Mr. Jones is uncomfortable in a small car requires the additional use of only common knowledge generalizations.

The explanation function of diagnostic propositions, and their closely related use in prediction, is a feature of such propositions that is of great importance in clinical diagnosis. This will be discussed in the following sections.

REFERENCES AND FOOTNOTES: CHAPTER 3

1. R B Price and Z. R. Vlahcevic, "Logical Principles in Differential Diagnosis," Ann Int Med, 75 (1971) 90.
2. Ibid, pp. 90-91.
3. Ibid, p. 894
4. R. C. Cabot, Differential Diagnosis (Philadelphia: W. B. Saunders, 1911), pp. 18-19.
5. G. L. Engle, "The Deficiencies of the Case Presentation as a Method of Clinical Teaching," New Eng J Med, 284, No. 1 (7 Jan., 1971), 22.New Eng J Med., 284, No. 1 (7 Jan, 1971), p22.
6. T. P. Almy, "Disorder of Motility," in Beeson and McDermott, (eds): Cecil-Loeb Textbook of Medicine.13th ed. Philadelphia: W. B. Saunders Co., 1971 , p. 1247.
7. Eddy, D., NEJM Vol 306 No. 21, May 27 1982, "The art of diagnosis." pp 1263-1268
8. Barrows, H.S. et al., Clinical and Investigative Medicine, Vol 5:1,"The clinical reasoning of randomly selected physicians in general medical practice." pp 49-55, 1982 , writing: "This tactic strongly resembles the hypothetico-deductive approach described for many years as the inquiry method of scientists," and "The physicians generate, on average, 5.5 hypotheses in each encounter..."
9. Stanley D.E. et al, Perspectives in Biology and Medicine, Vol 56, no. 2,(spring 2013) , "The Logic of Medical Diagnosis" pp 300-315 Referring to C. S. Peirce (1839-1914), the authors adopt the Peirce notion of "abduction,"(the forming of causal hypotheses).
10. Kassirer, J., Annals of Internal Medicine 1989; 110"Diagnostic Reasoning" pp 893-900 This author writes of causal reasoning, and also uses statistical data as well as subjective probabilities.

11. An exception, e.g., could be singular propositions with the same empirical content, or when the "derivative" proposition has less such content than the other, etc., depending on inferential rules.

12. As "feature" would generally be understood in clinical medicine; it may correspond to a complex property.

13. The disease "streptococcal pharyngitis" may be accompanied by variable amounts of inflammation ("pharyngitis"), or may occur in a "subclinical" form.

14. Examples of straightforward use of (1) (e.g., in the diagnosis of a "classic" case of "Cushing's syndrome") may be construed as resting on the assumption that nothing (known) other than the given "syndrome" could account for the features presented (a very good diagnostic criterion), an assumption which may in some cases be supported by available medical knowledge and theory. But as in the usual case this assumption is not reliable, as situations permitting such use of (1) are exceptional.

15. But it is not the case that there are one-to-one correlations between "syndromes" and their "etiologies" (certainly when these are construed as diseases) for a certain disease may only sometimes lead to a given "syndrome" (e.g., the "superior vena caval syndrome" in lung cancer), or may lead to altogether different syndromes (e.g., the "ectopic-ACTH syndrome" in lung cancer), and the same "syndrome," as conventionally defined, may conversely arise from different diseases (there are many obvious examples, including both "syndromes" mentioned in this paragraph).

16. "We will mention evidence only to establish only why diagnosis should trump evidence." Stanley DE & Campos DG, Op cit., p. 301

17. Remember also the famous maxim: "When possible treat the disease, not the symptoms."

18. The importance of these in disease definition has brought about major changes in modern medical nosology, broadening and deepening this from its concern with pathological anatomy. Many diseases as now

understood have no (or no <u>defining</u>) anatomic pathological changes, although the latter may occur as their <u>effects</u>.

19. Among reasons for a general rejection of operationalism is the insight encapsulated by K. Popper in the remark: "... *measurements presuppose theories.*" (<u>Conjectures and Refutations</u>, [New York and London: Basic Books, 1962], p.62) Italics original.

20. Not only is "sweetness of the urine" now not a necessary condition for this diagnosis, but neither is it any longer sufficient. For other (more recently defined) diseases are known to have the same manifestation (e.g., "renal glycosuria," "essential pentosuria," etc.), further reflecting the impact of theory on this diagnostic term.

21. Source: "Medicine.Nat.com," (Google), April 29, 2016

22. Consider the different theoretical implications but similar empiric conditions for use of "opening snap" and "S₃ heart sound," and the similarly problematic relations between "S₃ heart sound" and "S₄ heart sound."

CHAPTER 4

Explanation, Prediction and Medical Diagnosis

Introduction

Having seen that diagnostic propositions may serve an explanatory role in medicine, the nature of this role and its relevance to the diagnostic process will be discussed.

Medical explanation involving diagnostic propositions conforms, I will argue, to the most common and historical form of scientific explanation, as characterized by Carl Hempel: "A scientific explanation... may be regarded as a potential answer to a question of the form 'why is it the case that p?', where the place of 'p' is occupied by an empirical sentence detailing the facts to be explained."[1] For our purposes the empirical sentence, 'p' will attribute to a patient a certain property or state. This will ordinarily be a particular manifestation (a sign or symptom) of disease, but may at another level describe a disease state itself. Furthermore, such explanations will require use of empiric generalizations or law-like statements.[2]

On this account, it may in general be said that a certain manifestation of a patient's disease can be <u>explained</u> by means of a joint assertion of a diagnostic proposition (naming the patient) and at least one empiric law-like statement relating the event or processes referred to by the diagnostic predicate with the given manifestation. While it is not claimed that this is the only way in which the manifestation might be explained, it is the way that involves diagnostic propositions, with which we are concerned. In most cases, additional singular propositions and/or law-like statements will be required to complete the explanation. In any case, such an explanation requires some kind of <u>inference</u>, the detailed structure of which depends on the nature of the law-like statement(s) employed.[3-5]

Law Statements in Medicine

Several kinds of law-like statements are commonly used in medical diagnosis, explicitly or implicitly. Their major types will be outlined and discussed in the following sections. Special attention will be devoted to causal and closely related laws, the use of which provides helpful clues in an account of the diagnostic process.[6]

1.   <u>Functional laws</u>

These are mathematically precise and at least approximately true laws relating several variables, which may vary over certain continuous ranges. A well-known example of such a law in common use in clinical medicine relates the acidity (pH) of the blood to its carbon dioxide buffer system, as expressed in the so-called "Henderson-Hasselbach" equation:

$$pH = pK + \log (HCO_3-)$$

———

$$H_2CO_3$$

where the terms receive their usual chemical interpretations. Equations such as this rely heavily on physicochemical theory. This equation is of considerable value to clinical diagnosis for its theoretic terms occur in many places in medical science (alveolar $CO2$ diffusion, renal tubular bicarbonate transport, etc.). Laws such as this serve to quantitatively link terms within an established theoretical network.

2. Statistical Laws

It is commonly assumed that most or perhaps all the laws and generalizations in medical science are statistical. This view exaggerates our degree of ignorance. Worse, it is not consistent with the assumption common among medical scientists that phenomena at the level of nature covered by such laws are more likely to be causal (deterministic) than intrinsically statistical. More in keeping with this assumption and with ordinary clinical methods is the construal of most of the probabilistic laws in medicine as poorly formulated causal laws, in which there is incomplete specification of relevant causal conditions, rather than as laws that are irreducibly statistical. One may expect at least some of these to be replaced by ordinary causal laws with advances in medical knowledge.

The various ways in which statistical or otherwise probabilistic law statements that may serve in the proposed model of medical diagnosis will be examined.

3.   Tendency Laws

This term was proposed by R. Braithwaite, a well-known philosopher of science (England, 1900-1990), who characterizes these laws ("statements")[6] thus: "The peculiarity of a tendency statement is that it states that, if a thing is C, then, if it is also A it is also B, where 'If a thing is A it is also B' (i.e., Every A is B) is an ordinary scientific hypothesis, and C is an unspecified property."[7]

Historically, this concept goes back at least to John S. Mill (1806 – 1873), who wrote extensively on complex relations involving groups of multiple causes and effects in nature,[8] and was more recently advocated by Harold Kincaid in defense of social sciences.[9]

In Braithwaite's terminology, the ordinary causal law (assuming the statement true) "Every A is B" (or, If A then B) can be schematically represented:

(1) $A \rightarrow B$

The important characteristic of such a law is that every relevant feature of A is completely specifiable, and the occurrence of A is invariably followed by B. The qualification "relevant" is important to the workability of such a formulation in science. What is irrelevant are all those features of the world (if taken in toto, unspecifiable) the occurrences or non-occurrences of which have not been observed to affect the invariability of the association of A and B. (Of course, there may be good theoretic reasons for distinguishing what is relevant also). The physical sciences are fortunate in that it has proved relatively easy to specify relevant antecedent conditions, such as "A", sufficiently to formulate causal laws. The exchange of momentum between colliding billiard balls has proved, for example, to be highly immune to influence by features of the immediate environment (size of the table on which they are traveling, etc.), and even some features of the system itself (e.g., color of the balls).

The situation in medicine and biology has undoubtedly been more complex. There are few if any known associations of features in the human organism that are independent of other features of the organism, at least as these have so far been characterized in medical science. Nevertheless, causal type laws are common in modern medical science, and there are a great many tendency laws, which bear important resemblances to causal laws.

In Braithwaite's terminology, we may formulate a tendency law as follows:

(2) $C \dashrightarrow (A \dashrightarrow B)$

or by the logically equivalent expression:

(3) $(A \cdot C) \dashrightarrow B$

This may be read: "If A occurs, and C is present, then B occurs." An important point about such statements is that "C", part of the antecedent of this conditional, is not specifiable. Hence, the occurrence of an "A" not followed by "B" does not <u>refute</u> the tendency law, for such a case may be explained by the absence of "C". However, the association of "A" with "B" should be invariable (assuming the truth of (3)) within the classes of "A" and "B", which are subclasses of the class of "C."[10] It is another important feature of a tendency law that this restriction can be removed by specification of "C", thereby converting it to a corresponding causal law.11

It would be possible to cite many examples of tendency laws in use in clinical medicine. If "A" is taken to represent a disease, and "B" to represent any one of its manifestations, whenever their association is not invariable, as is commonly the case, the statement of their association may be viewed as at least a *prima facie* instance of a tendency law.

It is important at this point to distinguish statements that are tendency laws where "C" is altogether unspecifiable, from those that are rather elliptically formulated causal laws in which "C" is not completely unspecifiable but for certain purposes remains unspecified. These ideal types are clearly not always realized in fact, for it frequently happens that "C" is partially but not completely specifiable. The latter situation is especially apt to occur in areas of science experiencing rapid development, as is now the case in clinical medicine. Most tendency law statements associating diseases with their manifestations in use in clinical medicine—the obvious utility of such statements should be borne in mind—are in such transitional logical status, in which clinicians are able, if challenged, to more or less satisfactorily specify an appropriate "C". In these cases, the logic in the use of a tendency law may be made to resemble that of a causal law. It is in such use, furthermore, that tendency laws also serve a vital heuristic function (stimulating interest and investigation)12 in medical science, a function that would not readily be served by a merely statistical treatment of the association of A with B.[13]

Consider, for example, the association of the disease tuberculosis, with one of its manifestations, the positive tuberculin skin test. It is known that not every patient who has or has had tuberculosis ("A") will, if tested, exhibit a positive skin test ("B"). We may characterize this situation with the statistical assertion that a certain proportion of patients with A will exhibit B, or by the claim that there is a certain statistical probability of a given patient with A also having B. While such an assertion may be of primary (and perhaps exhaustive) interest to some (e.g., an epidemiologist) concerning the association of A with B, it falls far short of exhausting the clinician's interest in, or knowledge of, this association. For the clinician, who reasons causally, the association can be better characterized by a tendency law formulation:

(4) $(A \cdot C) \text{----} \rightarrow B$

where it is possible to partially specify "C" by statements such as the following:

(i)   The patient has a normal immune system. This hypothesis must (and can) be tested by independent means.

(ii) The patient does not have a <u>massive infection</u>. This hypothesis must (and can) be independently tested.

(iii) The skin test is done accurately, i.e., using fresh materials, proper technique, etc.

(iv) The patient has not received anti-tuberculous therapy.

"C" is sufficiently complex in this instance (and the above list is not intended to be complete) that any inference from "A" to "B" will require the use of several laws or generalizations (e.g., the non-occurrence of an inability to develop immunity to only one kind of antigen, the persistence of cellular immunity, etc.). Many of these are the objects of research. Enough is already known, however, that any patient with a history of established tuberculosis who satisfies conditions (i)--(iv) and yet failed to exhibit a positive tuberculin skin test might well become a subject of investigation. Such an occurrence would be seen by clinicians as demanding an <u>explanation</u> (the specification of previously unrecognized features of "C"), exemplifying the important heuristic (investigative) function in the use of a tendency law.

Of course, conditions such as (i)-(iv) are not always fulfilled, a fact that is connected to another important feature in the use of (3). For the failure of certain of these conditions (e.g., (i), in the present example) is itself an abnormality, providing evidence for the presence of some other disease that may have been unsuspected. Hence, a negative tuberculin skin test in a patient with a known history of tuberculosis provides, when conditions (ii)-(iv) are believed to obtain, evidence for the patient's having a disorder of the immunologic system. Accordingly, the tuberculin skin test has found use in testing for such diseases, as well as in the diagnosis of tuberculosis. Analogous considerations apply to the uses of the mumps skin test, and others, in which such secondary uses of the test in assessing immune system function have been at times more important than its primary one.

On the assumption that the partial or complete unspecifiability of "C" in a tendency law is only a matter of fact and not one of principle, a common working assumption in the use of such laws in medical science, it is clear from the proposition "If a thing is C then if it is also A it is also B" that a tendency law is thoroughly <u>causal</u> in its conception.[14] In such terms, a tendency law can be understood to represent the linking of "A" with "B" by means of a causal chain that is not complete, i.e., there are one or more points at which it may be (causally) interrupted. Schematically, the situation may be depicted thus:

$$C_1 \qquad C_2 \qquad C_n$$
$$\underline{\hspace{1cm}} \quad \underline{\hspace{1cm}} \quad \underline{\hspace{1cm}}$$

$$A \text{ -------- } A_1 \text{ --------------- } A_2 \text{ --------------- } A_n \text{ -------- } B$$

where A_1, A_2, ... etc. are intermediate events and C_1, C_2, ... etc. collectively specify "C". Every component of "C" is essential at some point in the causal chain for its progression toward "B".[15]

In general, I see this form of representation of more or less regular but not invariable empiric associations of interest in medicine as conforming far better in keep with clinical concepts and practices than any representation of such associations by only statistical means. In medical diagnosis or treatment, the occurrence of an "A" not followed by the expected occurrence of "B" is not usually accepted by the clinician as a matter of mere chance (unlike the non-disintegration of a particular atom of a known radioisotope during a certain time interval). For the clinician such an occurrence stimulates an attempt to answer the question "why?". This is in respect to our hypothetical tuberculosis patient, where a negative tuberculin skin test would lead to repeat skin testing, a re-examination of the evidence on which the alleged diagnosis was made, and a testing of the patient for other possible diseases that could interrupt the A ----→ B causal sequence. Hence, while the association of "A" with "B" may be known not to be invariable, the clinician tends to use the causal law, "A ----→ B", as though it were, and to conduct an educated search for an explanation when the expected association fails to hold.[16] While it is therefore not contended that statistical techniques may not be useful in relation to such associations, however, it is argued that these can in general be more satisfactorily represented in tendency law terms, and that the use of the latter in clinical medicine is logically akin to the use of ordinary causal laws. Within such a conceptual framework statistical techniques find, in fact, a natural place, as in the specification of normal intervals, which may be sometimes (not always) essential to the definition of such properties or events as "A" and "B". [17] However, it would be a mistake to conclude from these uses that such techniques comprise the clinician's conceptual framework itself.

4.   Causal Laws

Together with functional laws, which may be regarded as a mathematical form of causal laws (their logic of use in

medicine is similar), as converted tendency laws, where causally relevant antecedent conditions of an event have become
adequately specifiable, become like many other causal laws.
New causal and tendency laws are part of growth in medical
science, including cellular, and molecular and genetic
domains, among others.

An example of a well-known disease could be sickle-cell
anemia. During nearly half of the twentieth century, this
disease was understood in terms of abnormal red blood cells,
prone to fragility leading to anemia and other major signs
and symptoms. Diagnosis at that time depended largely on
microscopic examination of the blood, showing peculiar
sickle-like formed red cells. The proximal and deeper cause of
this disease was discovered by Linus Pauling in 1949, finding
the "substitution of a single valine residue for a glutamic acid
in each half molecule of hemoglobin."[18,19] This was more
recently discovered to be the effect of a single abnormal
gene, as summarized by Bunn: "a single base substitution in
the gene encoding the human B-globin subunit, with the
resulting replacement of B-6 glutamic acid by valine, leads
to the protean and devastating manifestations of sickle cell
disease."[20] The presence of the abnormal chemical, gene, and
hemoglobin molecules in this disease results in a predictable genetic pattern among carriers and patients affected
with this disease, converting a previous tendency law to an
ordinary causal law.[21] This progression also exemplifies the
heuristic (stimulus to discovery) role in causal reasoning.

While sickle-cell anemia still includes reference in its
definition to its familiar peripheral blood abnormalities, it
is equally certain that the theoretic genetic and molecular
abnormalities now figure in this definition and, correspondingly, in the diagnostic and other uses of the term. Clinicians

speak of sickle-cell disease, as such patients are not just anemic and genetic and molecular abnormalities are known to be more proximal causes in its many manifestations.

Other examples from clinical medicine of causal laws, or simply statements of invariable associations, could be offered. However, the matter need not be pursued here beyond recognizing the presence and important uses of such law-statements in modern clinical medicine.

REFERENCES AND FOOTNOTES: CHAPTER 4

1. C. G. Hempel, "Explanatory Incompleteness," in Brodbeck, <u>Readings in the Philosophy of the Social Sciences</u>, New York: The MacMillan Co. (1968) p. 407. The proviso would usually be added that the "potential answer" must contain reference only to events which are simultaneous with or antecedent to the event to be explained. The use of "teleological" explanation is infrequently encountered in modern clinical medicine (with the possible exception of psychiatry), although such explanation may sometimes serve a useful function in guiding or stimulating investigation.

2. A. Rosenberg op cit., p.27: "The empiricist account of causation holds that the relation of cause and effect obtains only when one or more laws <u>subsume</u> the events so related – that is, cover them as cases or instances of the operation of the law. Thus the initial or boundary conditions of the <u>explanans</u> cite the cause of the <u>explanandum</u> phenomenon, which are the effects of the boundary conditions according to the law mentioned in the <u>explananans</u>."

3. Not all such explanations will be "complete" in the ideal sense (cf. Hempel, ibid., pp. 401-11) of being fully explicit and specific; they may be "incomplete" in varying senses and degrees (following Hempel, they may be "elliptical" or "partial"). While such "incompleteness" affects the logical force of the explanation, it does not alter its general form.

4. DA Rizzi, and SA Pedersen, Theoretical Medicine 13:233-254 (1992) "Causality in medicine: Towards a theory and terminology.

5. It is clear that a diagnostic concept cannot be used to "explain" (in the above sense) those features of a disease that are its <u>defining characteristics.</u> Hence, the presence of "conjunctivitis" cannot be explained in the indicated manner by "Reiter's syndrome" (the common definition of which includes "conjunctivitis"). Logically problematic situations on our account may occur when such "manifest" defining characteristics

exist but are poorly specified. These situations are encountered less frequently as "syndromes" are replaced by disease concepts that are more etiologically, and more theoretically and precisely, defined. A "syndrome" may be said to "explain" the presence of its defining features in the weaker (psychological) sense of relieving the need for an explanation of these features by reference to other possible diseases (causes) in relation to which they are only "manifestations." Consider, e.g., the many diseases which may result in "conjunctivitis". Moreover, the "disease" versus "manifestation" relation often obtains and is explanatorily useful even for "syndromes," as "Reiter's syndrome" may be used in explanation of such other common features of this "disease" as various constitutional symptoms, mucocutaneous lesions, certain laboratory abnormalities, etc. In relation to an even simpler diagnostic concept, "wound," it is interesting to consider remarks by Hanson: "'The scar on his arm was caused by a wound...' Here 'wound' is an explanatory word..."; "Scars are what most wounds result in; hence it explains a man's scar to say that it was caused by a wound..." and "Similarly 'wound' explains the man's scar only against the implicit background of theory brought out here." (N R Hanson, Cambridge University Press, Cambridge, England (1965) "Patterns of Discovery." Pp55-57 This exemplifies the coupling of cause and effect empiric events in chain-like connections, a common phenomenon in medicine.

6. For present purposes I am calling such statements "laws." Arguments for and against doing so are not essential here.

7. Braithwaite, R.B., Scientific Explanation. 2nd edition, Harper and Row, New York and London, 1960

8. Nagel, E., The Hafner Library of Classics, Number 12 , Chapter x, "John Stuart Mill's Philosophy of Scientific Method" Hafner Publishing Co., New York pp 238-269

9. Kincaid, H., Readings in the philosophy of social science, Cambridge, Mass.: MIT Press, 1994, "Defending Laws in the Social Sciences" pp111-130. Note that the author uses the term "ceteris paribus" ("other

things being equal"), a different slant on unspecifiable conditionals but used much like "tendency" laws.

10. The success and apparent truth of any causal law may be similarly restricted and contingent, whether recognized or not, as in the laws of Newtonian physics.

11. Ibid. Cf. 10

12. "Heuristic" here, and elsewhere in this book, meaning that which stimulates interest and further investigation, and not a kind of "shortcut."

13. Cf. the following remarks by Hempel: "To the extent that a statement of individual causation leaves the relevant antecedent conditions, and thus also the requisite explanatory laws, indefinite it is like a note saying that there is a treasure hidden somewhere. Its significance and utility will increase as the location of the treasure is more narrowly circumscribed as the relevant conditions and the corresponding covering laws are made increasingly explicit. In some cases this can be done quite satisfactorily; the covering-law structure then emerges, and the statement of individual causal connection becomes amenable to test. When, on the other hand, the relevant conditions or laws remain largely indefinite, a statement of causal connection is rather in the nature of a program, or of a sketch, for an explanation in terms of causal laws; it might also be viewed as a "working hypothesis" which may prove its worth by giving new, and fruitful, direction to further research." (Aspects of Scientific Explanation [New York: The Free Press, 1965] pp. 349-350.)

14. It may sometimes be true that "C" is so complex as to make its complete specification impracticable now or in the foreseeable future. (Cf. in physics the dropping in air of leaves on a target.) That the outcomes of such processes are practically manageable only in statistical terms does not imply that the processes involved are not subject to causal laws. It may also be said that the uncertainty principle in quantum mechanics is not generally seen to be of importance in the formulation

of laws in biology and medical science. It is only these laws and their uses which are under consideration, and not the question which scientific laws (or their forms) are "ultimately" true. The latter question, unlike the former, is in my view scientifically unanswerable.

15. Practical difficulties in the specification of "C" should not be lost sight of in this schematization. Some components of "C" may correspond to many-valued or continuous variables, for example, whose causal relevance to "B" may be subject to threshold conditions, etc. (as in the "freshness" of tuberculin skin test materials). The assessment of their potential or actual realization in individual instances will be correspondingly complex.

16. Scriven, M. In Gardner P. (ed) Theories of History, The Free Press, Glencoe, Ill. (1959) "Truisms as the Ground for Historical Explanation" pp 465-467 In arguing the important role of such statements in causal explanations of individual occurrences, Scriven writes: "... statistical statements are too weak -- they abandon the hold on the individual case." The sense and extent in which this is true is clearly connected with the failure of such statements to satisfy the clinician, whose recurrent and overriding interest is the individual case.

17. Not all such properties in clinical medicine require statistics in their definition, for many of these are conceived in "all-or-nothing" terms (including many if not most "disease" concepts (e.g., malignant diseases, infectious diseases, lacerations, subdural hematomas, atrial fibrillation, etc.). Moreover, the use of statistics in the definition of a property does not imply that the property is subject only (if at all) to statistical laws, a belief which, as has been argued, would in any case be contrary to the usual assumptions of clinical scientists. It is interesting to note in this connection that while in the case of ordinary statistical variables rare events, or values, are permitted (in a sense, "predicted"), most "variables" in use in clinical medicine are not, in fact, so regarded. Hence, for example, a serum bilirubin concentration of 2.0 mg% (say), although only a few "standard deviations" from its statistical "mean"

value, in relation to which abnormal values are defined, would by most clinicians <u>never</u> be accepted as a mere "chance" variation, but would <u>always</u> be seen as a manifestation of some abnormal process, subject to some kind of causal explanation, which would routinely be sought. It is sometimes suggested that clinicians are naive and/or simply wrong in this. But I think that experience supports the clinician's view, and instead that interpretation and treatment of the serum bilirubin concentration, as in our example, theoretically subject to various causal mechanisms of control, in <u>merely</u> statistical terms is itself a mistake. Also subject to mistake would be any <u>a priori</u> assumptions, when it is treated statistically, concerning its actual distribution of values (useful determinations of which, as in "normal," will often depend on causal theory in the selection of reference classes), which may not conform to any ideal type. Whether or not the processes which are its determinants are "intrinsically statistical" is another question, but there are no compelling reasons for supposing that they are.

On the subject of the definition of "A" and "B" it should be observed that matters concerning the specification (and specifiability) of the "events" (which may be complex conditions) to which these refer are as important as those pertaining to "C" in the availability and use of tendency laws or analogously causal laws. The "availability" of a generalization concerning an association of such events will in general vary inversely, and its "empiric content" directly, with the exactness and completeness of their specification, and its usefulness in science will to some degree reflect its empiric content (assuming it is true). But the matter is by no means so simple, as natural phenomena to not always neatly conform to the conceptual idealizations of science. Even in physics requirements for exactness and completeness in the specification of "events" must not be too stringent, but must rather be "optimized" (e.g., by means of various simplifying assumptions) for the applicability and even the testability of the hypothetical laws of association. In medicine, while the complex phenomena as are referred to, for example, by most disease concepts which may be only inexactly and incompletely specified (or specifiable), such concepts have ample company in this regard, and may be nonetheless useful in empiric laws and generalizations.

18. H. E. Sutton H., "Human Hereditary and its Cytologic Bases," in J. Stanbury, J. Wyngaarden, and D. Frederickson, eds., The Metabolic Basis of Inherited Disease, 2nd ed. (new York and London: McGraw Hill, 1966), p.55.

19. Bunn, M. F., NEJM, September 11, 1997, "Pathogenesis and Treatment of Sickle Cell Disease" p 762

20. Bunn, M. F., Ibid., p762

21. A justification of this terminology is not important here, but I believe it to be correct. The stated association is universal, linked into a network of other laws and theory in medical science, supports the use of counterfactual conditional statements, etc.

CHAPTER 5

Models of Explanation

Many of the complex and controversial issues relating to explanation in science are not within the scope of our topic, nor is their discussion essential to its purposes. For these purposes it will, however, be useful to adopt and examine two explanation schemas embodying what is commonly called the "covering law" concept of scientific explanation. This widely known view has received its classic and perhaps fullest expression by Carl Hempel.[1-4] The relation of these schemas to explanation and prediction in clinical medicine, and of these latter to the diagnostic process, will be examined and discussed. It will be necessary in this to probe again the function of various types of medical law-statements in these schemas. Consideration of medical examples will be seen to bear both on clinical diagnosis and on some alternative views of scientific explanation.

In Hempel's terminology, the two models pertinent to our task are the deductive-nomological (D-N) and the inductive-statistical (I-S) models.

1.　　The Deductive-Nomological Model

Normal form

This model is un-problematically applicable only in cases where an explanation requires the use of only causal type laws (or, if there is terminological dispute, "laws of invariable association"). Following Hempel,[5] the logical structure of such an explanatory scheme can be represented as follows:

(1)　　($C_1, C_2, ... C_K$ Statements of antecedent conditions)

Logical

Deduction

$L_1, L_2, ... L_r$ General Laws　　　　Explanans

E Description of the empirical　　Explanandum

As indicated in the diagram the explanans consists of a variable number each of general laws (in this context, causal) and statements of antecedent conditions. The conjunction of these statements provides via a deductive inference a statement "E" describing the event to be explained (the explanandum). The truth of the explanans thus logically guarantees the truth of "E", whereas, of course, the truth of "E" provides no such assurance of the truth of the explanans (although it may be thereby in some sense "confirmed"). If "E" is false, on the other hand, at least one of the statements contained in the explanans must be false. Moreover, the same statements (and argument form) used in the explanation of past events can be used in the prediction of similar events in the future, with the same truth relations holding between the prediction and its premises. How does this schema apply to medical diagnosis?

In the diagnostic situation, we see that the diagnostic proposition must function as one of the statements of antecedent conditions. Conjoined with other such statements, and at least one causal law, "L," we can where this model is applicable deduce a statement "E" describing some (other) empirical phenomenon "e."

Consider the example of a patient with sickle-cell disease. A general account of the deduction of, say, "Mr. Jones has sickling of his red cells" from "Mr. Jones has sickle-cell disease" would require the use of various other statements of antecedent conditions (e.g., Mr. Jones has not recently received an exchange transfusion) and general laws (e.g., physico-chemical laws pertaining to the sickling test procedure, exchange transfusions, etc.). In practice, however, most of these are accepted tacitly[6] and the argument is presented in a condensed form:

2.   C1: Mr. Jones has sickle-cell disease

         L1: Every person with sickle-cell disease has abnormal red blood cells that under certain (specifiable) conditions "sickle." Conclusion: Mr. Jones has abnormal native red blood cells.

         An important logical point in the general account is that the non-occurrence of "e" implies the falsity of at least one of the statements in the explanans. In conformity with the use of the simplified argument (2), the clinician would ordinarily accept the non-occurrence of "e" as falsifying the diagnostic proposition "Cl". However, this will not always be the case, for it must be remembered, as the clinician recognizes, that the condensed version (2) is a simplification at the expense of some correctness of a more general deduction. Some of the tacitly assumed laws and (especially) statements of antecedent conditions may be false. The same considerations would apply to an analogous deduction involving hemoglobin electrophoresis, an example which might better avoid any factual quibble and in which the need for various other law statements may be more obvious.

Using this more general deductive scheme, in a given case of non-occurrence of an expected "e", a clinician must therefore reject at least one of the following:

(i)   the diagnostic proposition (hypothesis) "C_1".
(ii)   the law "L_1".
(iii) one of the tacitly assumed laws L_2, L_3, ... etc.
(iv)   one of the tacitly assumed statements of antecedent conditions.

Confronted with this situation, the clinician is in fact quite _free_ to choose between these alternatives, and her/his choice will depend on its context. She/he will in general be reluctant to reject those laws or generalizations that she/he believes to be well established. Her/his rejection of one or more of the statements of antecedent conditions, including the diagnostic hypothesis, will depend on her/his degree of confidence in these propositions (among them will often be statements that the patient has or does not have some other disease(s)). Finally, she/he may reject the allegedly contrary evidence "not-E", depending on all of the above and on his confidence in her/his own or others observations and, in

particular, the reliability of testing data. The sickling phenomenon, for example, may have been misread. More will be
said on this later.

Numerous other examples could be given of situations
in clinical medicine permitting use of deductive arguments
of the kind illustrated. Many of these would be variously
subject, however, to a criticism that has been made of the
deductive-nomological model, which therefore needs to be
considered. A point for attack on the model can be brought
out by means of an example.

Consider the following deductive argument:

C1: Mr. Smith has had a total gastrectomy

L1: Every person who has a total gastrectomy has
defective vitamin B12 absorption (if untreated).

E: Mr. Smith, untreated, has defective vitamin
B$_{12}$ absorption.

This argument could be used in practice, for example to
infer from Mr. Smith's normal vitamin B$_{12}$ absorption that
he has not had a total gastrectomy. Again, this argument is a
simplified version of a more general deductive scheme that
would include other statements of antecedent conditions, for
example that Mr. Smith is not receiving exogenous intrinsic
factor, a protein. Law statements that human intrinsic factor
is secreted in biologically significant amounts only in the
stomach, that it is essential in the transport of vitamin B$_{12}$
across the intestinal mucosa, etc. (such laws may be said,
incidentally, to explain "L$_1$", which is derivable from them).

Unfortunately, "L$_1$" is not, as it is written, quite true. It
would be made more correct by substitution of the phrase

"soon after the operation" for its second occurrence of "has." For there may be a certain temporal lag between total gastrectomy and the appearance of defective vitamin B12 absorption, the duration of which cannot be exactly specified. It will depend on, among other things, which test procedures are used for vitamin B_{12} absorption, etc. Such an amendment of "L_l" would, however, invalidate the argument as presented. Moreover, while in this example the criteria for attribution of the property "defective vitamin B_{12} absorption" (as well as for "total gastrectomy") are adequately specifiable (given available test procedures), this will not be as true for some other properties of interest in clinical medicine (e.g., weakness, emaciation, etc.). Vagueness in such terms will add to the difficulties in the formulation and use of empiric generalizations in which they occur.

Such problems are not peculiar to clinical medicine, but are found throughout science. Noting the pervasiveness of such problems in formulating true universal laws, even in the physical sciences, for example, the inaccuracies in the various gas laws, and the requirement for such laws in the deductive account, some philosophers have advocated a wider scope of explanation, including various pragmatic senses of this term.[7] It is not necessary here to make the claim that the covering law model explicates the sole legitimate sense of explanation or prediction in science or in everyday events. However, it is pertinent to question the seriousness to our account of other views such as those mentioned above, and the strength of the covering-law model to an account of explanation and prediction in clinical medicine.

For this purpose, it must first be recognized, as Hempel points out, that empiric generalizations refer not to individual events, but to events of certain kinds. Conjoined, however, with appropriate singular statements, and perhaps with other general statements, such a generalization may serve in the inferential derivation of a sentence describing the occurrence of an event of a particular kind. An <u>individual event</u> can then be explained (or predicted) only in the sense that it is, in Hempel's words (and italics his), "the <u>occurrence of a particular instance of a given kind of event</u>,"[10] i.e., that it satisfies generally accepted criteria for application of a given empiric characterization. Now the occasions of truth as well as applicability of an empiric generalization so construed will depend on, among other things, what requirements for descriptive exactness and completeness are met in its characterization of the (kinds of) events mentioned. A generalization that might fail under one such set of requirements may be universally true, and not necessarily trivial or useless, when reformulated to relax these requirements.

It is apparent that Hempel and Scriven[9] differ in respect to what such requirements they deem reasonable in relation to scientific laws and their uses. Hempel, for instance, gives the following explanation as an example of what can be subsumed under the <u>deductive nomological</u> model: "In his book, <u>How We Think</u>, John Dewey[11] describes a phenomenon he observed one day while washing dishes. Having removed some glass tumblers from the hot suds and placed them upside down on a plate, he noticed that soap bubbles emerged from under the tumblers' rims, grew for a while, came to a standstill, and finally receded into the tumblers. Why did this happen? Dewey outlines an explanation to this effect: Transferring the tumblers to the plate, he had trapped cool air in them; that air was gradually warmed by the glass, which initially had the temperature of the hot suds. This led to an increase in the volume of the trapped air, and thus to an expansion of the soap film that had formed between the plate and the tumblers' rims. But gradually, the glass cooled off, and so did the air inside, and as a result, the soap bubbles receded."[11]

Given (in Hempel's terms) the "explanandum phenomenon" (the formation, growth, and recession of soap bubbles) and "certain explanatory facts" consisting of "particular facts and... uniformities expressible by means of general laws," Hempel goes on to say, "If we imagine the various explicit or tacit explanatory assumptions to be fully stated, then the explanation may be conceived as a deductive argument of the form ... [D-N]."[12]

It is obvious that the workability of a deductive account in this example depends on there being only (not finer than) a <u>rough</u> characterization in the explanandum sentence of the phenomena to which it pertains. In an instance of the indicated antecedent kind—placing a hot sudsy tumbler upside down on a plate, the occurrence of a soap film beneath its rim, etc.—the formation thereupon of bubbles along the tumbler's outer rim, their initial growth followed by standstill and eventual recession, or some such rough characterization, is the <u>kind</u> of phenomenon to be explained. That this <u>kind</u> of phenomenon can be deduced, given the explanatory facts mentioned, seems clear. Equally clear, however, would be the dubious deducibility in relation to the same example, given the same—or any available—set of explanatory facts of a kind of phenomenon whose characterization would meet stricter requirements for exactness and completeness (e.g., in the number of bubbles formed, the location, time of appearance, rate of growth, maximum size, rate of recession, and moment of disappearance of each bubble, their color, shape, bursting, etc.). While <u>some</u> additional detail in an explanandum sentence may <u>sometimes</u> be purchased by refinement of the explanans, there will always be a point beyond which this becomes impracticable or impossible.[13] But while many such details may be provided, e.g., as in the bubble's biographies (which may be expanded ad infinitum), are not <u>deductively</u> inferable from such laws, initial conditions, etc. Many would accept this as a kind of scientific explanation, however, fitting in a "C" class depending on its details, given its likely rough character.

It is further apparent that the practical adequacy of an explanatory (or predictive) scheme in a given situation will hinge on the adequacy of the logically supported deductive or probabilistic explanandum-sentence, and that this will depend on the extent of the latter's descriptive detail in relation to what is <u>required</u> of it. It is a question, so to speak, of whether the descriptive net of the explanandum sentence so supported is sufficiently fine to capture at least the particular matters of interest in the given case. The answer to the factual question whether covering-law explanations (and predictions) are in this sense commonly accepted as adequate seems to me to be clearly affirmative.[14]

Take another appraisal of the bubble example. It would seem far easier to imagine situations in which the appropriate (needed or desired) characterization of such phenomena is of just the rough kind suggested than of a descriptively finer kind. Commonplace situations bearing an analogy to the example might include, for example, the storage of dangerous gases, places where the integrity of a seal is of concern, etc. Such a rough characterization will be satisfiable by a greater variety of possible facts than a more detailed one, the difference however being one of degree. It may alternatively be said to determine fewer empiric criteria for its inapplicability (omitting above, e.g., bubble color), and to determine these less exactly than would a more detailed description. Its applicability may permit aspects of interest a certain <u>range</u>, which may be closed either more exactly (at least one bubble forms after time "t₀") or less exactly (within a minute or so). But clearly excluded, for example, would be the first formation of bubbles at "t0 plus one hour, a phenomenon that would call for another explanation. What is then more important to the use of an empiric characterization than whether the permitted ranges of its aspects of concern are wide or narrow is whether they are <u>sufficiently</u> well determined to permit general agreement on the occasions of its applicability. What will be sufficient detail, in exactness and completeness, for such agreement will depend on how things are; it is an empiric matter of how much (if any) overlapping there is between the varieties of facts so characterized as a particular <u>kind</u> of phenomenon and those characterized differently. (Cf. sufficient conditions for uses of "Volkswagen" and "Ford," etc.) For a <u>kind</u> of phenomenon to form a useful concept, such agreement must at least obtain in typical cases in relation to which borderline cases, which may exist also for detailed descriptions, can be understood. Given such agreement—can it be doubted in the bubble example?—an empiric characterization (rough or fine) can find a useful place in the language of science.

These considerations have an obvious relevance in clinical medicine, where empiric concepts based on what have been called "rough characterization" of phenomena as <u>kinds</u> are the rule. Such concepts would include most diseases, signs, symptoms, and clinical test interpretations, e.g., positive sickle-cell test, positive tuberculin skin test, defective vitamin B12 absorption, etc. Phenomena of interest in medicine are usually not more than roughly quantifiable, in terms like "mild," "severe," "acorn-sized," "tightly-stenotic," etc. Even where relatively exact measurement is possible (e.g., in serum enzyme values), the range in which a value lies is generally as important in diagnosis as the exact value itself. However, by means requiring only such various degrees of exactness, clinical medicine has yet been able to differentiate many important, and importantly different, kinds of phenomena to study their inter-relations and to formulate generalizations concerning their universal or probabilistic associations. That the characterization of phenomena explained or predicted by arguments involving the use of such general statements will contain a corresponding inexactness does not affect the structure of such arguments. Moreover, the inexactness involved is often of little practical consequence.

Consider, for example, the following general statements, which, with the satisfaction of appropriate and specifiable initial and boundary conditions (including the absence of medical intervention), would be accepted by most clinicians as universally true of human organisms:

S_1: Continuous ventricular fibrillation is followed soon by death.
S_2: Saddle embolism with bilaterally complete pulmonary arterial occlusion is followed soon by death.
S_3: Acute bilateral renal tubular necrosis is followed soon by abnormal levels of serum creatinine.
S_4: Total gastrectomy is followed soon by defective vitamin B_{12} absorption.

There is obvious inexactness in the criteria for application of all the non-logical terms in these statements. Difficulties in the specification of exact criteria for "death," for example, have stirred controversy, e.g., in decisions for organ transplantation. But it is also clear that there are criteria for application of this term whose sufficiency would command general agreement; there is a point beyond which doubt is unreasonable. Analogous considerations apply to the other descriptive terms and phrases in these statements, each of which for clinicians has criteria for use that are similarly agreed to be <u>sufficient</u>. In relation to their <u>typical</u> uses, the fringe inexactness in these characterizations may be entirely irrelevant.

Further inexactness in S_1-S_4 is contained in the word "soon." The degree of this inexactness is quite comparable between S_1-S_2 ("within minutes") and between S_3-S_4 ("within days). It reflects the most exactly predictable time required for an organism to pass (via a causal pathway) from one state to another. Recall for comparison the bubble example, or processes involving conditions of dis-equilibrium in physics.) While there may again be difficulty concerning the exact temporal interval <u>necessary</u> to the truth of a given universal statement, there will yet be an interval that could be exactly specified if it mattered; e.g., "within ten minutes" for S_1-S_2, or "within ten days" for S_3-S_4, generally accepted as <u>sufficient</u> for this purpose.

Although the asserted relationship between states of the organism may be only probabilistic at times, much outside this range, or in otherwise fringe situations where attribution of a state is uncertain, conditions sufficient for use of the universal statement may be well understood, permitting if needed at least a <u>safe</u> specification of its scope. Construal of the general statement under such conditions as probabilistic would seem in general less reasonable or correct than a construal of borderline cases as probabilistic in the light of their location in the inexact fringe of a true law-statement's scope.

That accepted universal generalizations are not always available, or where available are not always clearly applicable is beside the point. The point is rather that even in clinical medicine, where much is inexact, such generalizations are abundant and important. It is inessential whether statements like S_1-S_4 should be called "laws," although in their expression of causal uniformities between empiric phenomena it is reasonable to do so. They are in any case <u>law-like</u> statements, derivatives of more general and increasingly more theoretic statements of causal associations in medicine, which may usefully serve in condensed forms of deductive medical explanation and prediction.

The divergence of this account from Scriven's and Kuhn's earlier analyses[15,16] depends importantly on a difference in construal of what <u>kinds</u> of phenomena can be, and are in fact, properly referred to by scientific law statements. It is claimed here that such kinds of phenomena in medical science comprise a certain variety of possible or actual facts, permitting, for example, a measured value (sufficiently determinate) relative to a certain latitude or range. For example, in relation to the abnormal features exhibited by the red blood cells of persons with sickle cell disease (in morphology, hemoglobin solubility, electrophoresis, genetics, etc.), quantitative detail (as in the exact proportion of red cells of a particular detailed form) is neither implicit in nor essential to their characterization as kinds of phenomena. It <u>might</u>, of course, have been the case that these general features in such persons would merge gradually with those of persons without this disease, but they don't. Their commonly accepted characterization as <u>kinds</u> of phenomena therefore reflect important natural differentiations, and permit study of the associations between these and other kinds of phenomena (e.g., persons with sickle cell disease have a propensity to develop symptoms under conditions of low oxygen tension, as in mountain climbing). Law-like statements of such associations are of profound importance in medical explanation and prediction. This is not to say that more exact laws are not useful in medicine (cf. the Henderson-Hasselbach equation), or that they may not <u>sometimes</u> be preferable to non-mathematical laws (they may not always be preferable, as if very cumbersome), but only that mathematical exactness is not essential to the argumentative—even deductive—uses of empirical law statements.[17]

Inexactness in medicine tends to surround the natural history (evolution) of diseases, including a patient's signs and symptoms, whereas modern imaging and laboratory tests provide relatively exact results. Nonetheless, inexactness can be difficult also in these and other—including physical—sciences, where discrepancies between exact values deduced from laws and singular statements and exact measured values are the rule. However, the importance attached by some in criticism of the deductive model is exaggerated. If an explanation is construed as an attempted answer to a "why?" question, then an approximate answer is quite likely the best that is possible in a complex world with an imperfect science. It is unreasonable to ask for absolute precision. A demand for an explanation why some aspect of an event is exactly what it is measured to be in extremely fine detail is one I can imagine no form of explanation in present day science would be consistently able to conform. However, this is no more fatal to what is accepted as adequate in scientific explanation than is the impossibility of an exactly correct description of such an aspect (in values to, say, nn decimal places) fatal to acceptable scientific description. Discrepancies between inferred and measured values will often reflect just such descriptive inaccuracies, and in at least some cases will be amenable to statistical analysis.[18] On the other hand, laws may sometimes be unacceptably inaccurate in their deductive uses. That this is commonly taken to imply a need for better (more accurate) laws supports the deductive model of their explanatory and predictive uses in science.

Rosenberg and others[19,20] bring up again the role of idealization in science, including the physical sciences (e.g., point source, perfect sphere, homogenous solid, ideal gases, etc.), where characterizations of phenomena as "kinds" are satisfiable by a variety of possible or actual facts. This may be true even at relatively fundamental levels, as is apparent in progress and controversy concerning the make-up of elementary particles. However, for example, while it may be the case that not all members of a class of particles still understood by many to be elementary are in fact identically constituted, the importance of their study as a discrete kind of phenomenon in relation to other such kinds is not lost in those common contexts—including nuclear medicine and proton radiation therapy—where their elementary characterization (omitting further details) is taken as sufficient. Law statements asserting associations of such kinds of phenomena will embody corresponding inexactness. While this will be transmitted by arguments involving the use of these statements in explanation or prediction, the typically deductive structure of such arguments is again unaffected. That re-characterizations of "effect-phenomena" (e.g., in more detail), often resulting from observed discrepancies in certain situations between calculated and measured values, typically form the basis for re-characterization of their antecedent conditions to further support the claimed deductive structure of their argumentative relations.

In short, inexactness affects the practical adequacy of a deductive explanation or prediction only insofar as it affects the determination whether relevant aspects of an individual event in question do or do not fall within the accepted purview of the kind [21] of phenomenon characterized in the logically supported explanandum sentence. The element of judgement involved in this determination is far less damaging to the deductive account than some have claimed, for there are many obvious examples of universal generalizations in medicine, as well as in physical sciences, in relation to whose common uses this judgement is entirely unproblematic, in spite of varying degrees of fringe inexactness in their scope.

The universal generalizations accepted, however tentatively, as true in medicine are thus importantly different from either tendency laws or probability statements. Hempel's deductive-nomological model provides the best general means for an explication of the deductive uses of such statements in medical explanation and prediction. This model is also helpful in explicating the uses of tendency laws in medicine, as will be considered in the next section. First, however, a few comments about the earlier statements, S_1 - S_4, are of interest.

Boundary and antecedent conditions were called only "specifiable" above. These conditions must be emphasized. Boundary conditions have to do with environment and context. Antecedent conditions have to do with history of a patient (in other sciences, object or phenomena), whether in investigative or practical uses. Such conditions are either assumed or carefully specified. Either way, such conditions are of fundamental importance. In clinical medicine, these conditions vary greatly with the patient context. Regarding statement S_1, for example, boundary conditions would include having a crash cart of appropriate drugs, cardioverter, etc., nearby. Antecedent conditions for this patient would include her/his cardiac history (previous or new myocardial infarction, heart failure, previous arrhythmias, etc.), and not only these, since her/his entire medical history, along with patient values and wishes, are important too. The variety of these conditions and their particular facets challenge the clinician's observations, medical knowledge, and judgment, supporting the axiom, "treat every patient as an individual case." This theme will be revisited.

3. The deductive–nomological model in relation to tendency laws.

As discussed earlier, tendency laws in medicine express associations of empiric phenomena that are known not to be invariable, or are at least not firmly believed to be invariable. In this they clearly differ from law statements, which are accepted as genuine universals.[23] In our previous terminology, such an association of "A" with "B", may be formulated in tendency-law terms as "$(A \cdot C) \rightarrow B$", where "C" represents a condition (or set of conditions) that is unspecifiable, or not completely specifiable. But that "C" may be partially specifiable is important as the strength of the association of "A" with "B" will commonly be known to vary with the assessed presence of more or less well specifiable causally relevant conditions. Under some such reasonably specifiable conditions, the association may be practically invariable. While the associations expressed by tendency laws might correctly be called probabilistic, the construal of such laws in simple statistical terms is misleading in respect to their underlying causal associations and the manner of their use in clinical medicine. In this, at least many such statements are treated as quasi-universals,[24] whose logic of use, and its methodological import, can best be understood in relation to the deductive-nomological model.

Consider the variable association of tuberculosis infection with a positive tuberculin skin test. The quasi-universal ("S_T") phrase, "all patients with a history of untreated tuberculosis will exhibit a positive tuberculin skin test," is used in many contexts in the explanation or prediction of the outcome of a particular skin test. Successful instances of such uses are accepted as a matter of course, as with a normal universal, but in its failures resides a difference.

The details of this difference can be brought out by noting that such uses of this quasi-universal represent a simplification of a more general (in this case, quasi-) deductive account.[25] The more general scheme would contain other general statements and other statements of initial and boundary conditions (e.g., the patient is not treated with immunosuppressant drugs). These other singular statements will comprise those elements in "C" that are reasonably well specifiable within a given state of knowledge. In the case of a tendency-law, this specificity will remain in some measure incomplete. A failure of the quasi-universal "S_t" will not be readily dismissed by the clinician as a matter of enigmatic chance, in spite of the imperfections in the given association. In such cases he will rather bring to mind the more general (quasi-) deductive account, and in relation to this consider the same set of options as were discussed earlier; the non-occurrence of an expected event "e" may be attributed to <u>any</u> of the singular or law-like statements used in the deduction. Attribution of the failure to what is causally inexplicable (chance) will as a rule be the clinician's <u>last resort</u>, for in relation to clinical diagnosis and treatment it is the alternative of <u>least importance</u>. Recognizing that the search may not always succeed, the clinician will nevertheless routinely investigate those partially specifiable elements in "C" that <u>might</u> causally account for failure of the (quasi-) deduction. In diagnostically problematic cases, certainly, it is only after a thorough search of this kind that such a failure would be attributed, and then usually only <u>tentatively</u>, to what might be considered the unresolved remnant of chance in the tendency law. This remnant is neither accurately quantifiable nor static, but changes regularly with new knowledge and techniques of clinical testing. The important investigative functions of tendency laws in clinical medicine, and the inadequacy of their construal as statistical, are again apparent.

It is inessential to the methodological correctness and importance of such uses of tendency laws as quasi-universals in medical diagnosis that they be associated with a numerically high probability. What is important to these uses is that elements of "C" are partially specifiable. What is more specifiable in "C" is of most immediate interest in the <u>application</u> of a tendency law in individual diagnostic contexts. However, the elucidation of what is less specifiable in "C", of most immediate concern in clinical investigation, takes place largely in the <u>same contexts</u> (the diagnosis and treatment of persons with disease), bringing out the close connection between these aspects of clinical medicine.

The use in medicine of ordinary statistical statements, which may include those tendency laws where there is little understanding of causally relevant conditions in "C", will be considered in the framework of an inductive-statistical model of explanation.

4.   Inductive-Statistical model.

Induction can be used in explanation (or prediction) in situations of uncertainty. It is commonly used in sciences, including clinical medicine. It is also used a great deal in ordinary human activities, given the myriad complexities of the world around us. It generally leads to probabilistic (uncertain) conclusions. How can such reasoning be grounded and formalized?

As discussed in chapter 2, logicians classify probability theory into two perspectives: objective and subjective.

Objective

Objective probability rests on counting ratios of empiric events, often runs sufficiently long to satisfy statistical rules (theorems and laws). Mathematical statisticians and logicians dealing with such experimental and theoretical long-run events are commonly called frequentists.

The Frequentist model

There is a practical sense in which individual events may be said to be explained or predicted by the use of statistical statements.

Following a long history in this vein, dealing particularly with gambling (games of chance), Hempel, a logical empiricist, and others have explicated the inductive-statistical ("I-S") model of scientific explanation and prediction.[26-28] This model has been used in explanation and prediction in clinical medicine.

Utilizing a frequency interpretation Hempel summarizes thus:[29]

"Let F be a given kind of random experiment and G a possible result of it; then the statement that $p(G,F) = r$ means that in a long series of repetitions of F, it is practically certain that the relative frequency of the result G will be approximately equal to r,"[30] Hempel adopts from Cramer[31] the following two corollaries of this interpretation:

"(C.1) "If $1- p(G,F) < \varepsilon$, where ε is some very small positive number, then if random experiment F is performed one single time, it is practically certain that result G will occur."

"(C.2) "If $p(G,F) < \varepsilon$, where ε is some very small positive number, then if random experiment F is performed one single time, it is practically certain that result G will not occur."

Examining the statistical problem of explaining (or predicting) the result of an individual draw (D) of a ball from an urn in which most (999/1000) balls are white (W), Hempel utilizes corollary (C.1) in formulating the following logical schema.[32]

$$1 - p(W,D) < .0011$$

Dd
_____(makes practically certain)

_____

Wd

Hempel then formalizes a more general schema thus:

$$p(G,F) = r$$

$$\frac{\dfrac{F_i}{\quad\quad\quad\quad\quad\quad}}{G_i} \quad (r)$$

where the explanans "confers the logical probability r upon the explanandum statement."[33]

As it is given that statistically-based explanations and predictions of individual events have a place in science, it would seem that some such account is needed of the rationale for these uses. Several aspects of Hempel's account as they relate to clinical medicine will be discussed.

The Accuracy of "r"

The identification of the logical probability "r" holding between such explanans and its explanandum statements with an appropriate statistical probability ("p(G,F)") I see as sound. Problematic in practice, however, is the specification of an appropriate statistical probability. Hempel's discussion centers around a construal of "p(G,F) = r" in terms of "quantitatively definite statistical laws."[34] This requirement would often be too stringent in medical science, for probabilistic explanations in medicine are commonly offered and supposed to be adequate in contexts much more complex than drawing from an urn of balls (with a known distribution of colors) where statistical probabilities invoked are not known in more than rough quantitative terms. This is commonplace in clinical medicine, where the explanatory use of such a statistical probability does not even require that it be numerically high (see below). On the other hand, not every statistical probability—precise or rough—is <u>appropriate</u> for use in a potential individual patient. This will be discussed in a later chapter.

The Range of "r"

Hempel says, "an argument of this kind will count as explanatory only if the number 'r' is fairly close to 1. But it seems impossible, without being arbitrary, to designate any particular number, say .8, as the minimum value of the probability 'r' permissible in an explanation."[35]

While there should be little disagreement with the latter part of this quotation, and while the former part may work in some situations, it is not workable in many explanatory contexts in clinical medicine.

As deductive explanations are generally preferable to probabilistic ones, so are those probabilistic explanations with (in Hempel's terms) a high associated probability ("r") generally preferable to those with a low associated probability.[36-37] This will be especially so in contexts where attention is less confined to a more-or-less definite set of possible (sometimes probabilistic) causes of an event to be explained than in typical situations of clinical diagnosis (the difference should not be taken too strictly). The present account varies from Hempel therefore in allowing the adequacy of probabilistic explanations a freer range over their associated probabilities, allowing also that the force of such explanations will in many contexts diminish with a low associated probability.

Relevant Evidence

It is clear that in probabilistic medical explanation some requirement dealing with the use of total relevant evidence is needed for the acceptability (or adequacy) of such explanations. This condition is not a theorem but a methodological rule that applies not only in parts of medical reasoning but also in other sciences.[38-40] However necessary as this rule is to the adequacy of inductive-statistical explanation, it is ambiguous and in clinical reasoning not generally <u>sufficient</u>, as the requirement stipulates only <u>available</u> evidence. As clinicians well know (and medical students early discover), requirements for adequacy in probabilistic explanation in medical diagnosis tend to be more stringent than this, demanding not only that all available evidence (whatever the given knowledge situation happens to be) known to be relevant be taken into account, but also that this account should actually include all (or as much as is judged needed and justified by considerations of risk, cost, seriousness of disease, etc.) information known to be of <u>potential</u> relevance to the explanandum event.

Hempel exemplifies the importance of relevant evidence in the case of a hypothetical patient, Mr. Jones, with a streptococcal infection. Suppose the patient is treated with penicillin and fails to recover. Another patient (Mr. Smith) is introduced, an octogenarian with a weak heart and a similar infection, and he fails treatment with penicillin. Are these patients likely to be similarly worked up (interviews, examinations, and testing)? Not likely. Many factors can cause or invite infection, and many others can affect antibiotic potency (e.g., fluid and electrolyte imbalance, wounds, immune function, leucocyte response, location of the infection, abscess formation, other drugs, etc.) of known potential relevance to the assumed outcome in such cases. The nature of the influence of such complex factors in relation to a given explanandum-event, of major interest to the clinician, is of course not here in question; what is material is rather that the adequacy of <u>any</u> probabilistic explanation in clinical medicine is dependent on an <u>appropriately comprehensive</u> assessment of information of known <u>potential</u> relevance to the explanandum-event. Bear in mind that pertinent negative findings, e.g., that Mr. Jones does not have a weak heart, are of comparable importance in medical reasoning to their corresponding positives.[41]

Like the requirement for the practical adequacy of probabilistic explanation in clinical medicine that all evidence in a certain knowledge situation known to be relevant to the explanandum-event be taken into account, the further requirement for such adequacy that the knowledge situation utilized must meet a certain appropriate standard of completeness in respect to information of known potential relevance to the event in question is not a theorem of inductive logic (or statistical theory), but is rather a <u>methodological principle</u>. Of major importance in clinical method, this principle again modifies the applicability of Hempel's inductive-statistical model of explanation in medicine. For the requirement that any <u>adequate</u> probabilistic explanation of clinical events be relatively complex in respect to its information content further diminishes the plausibility of interpreting the logical relation between this and the explanandum-event as one that "...invokes quantitatively statistical laws,"[42] or is itself quantitatively exact. Suppose, for example, that we are concerned with the probable (either explanatory or predictive) outcome of therapy in a Mr. Smith who is a poorly-nourished octogenarian with fairly good cardiac function but with moderate leucopenia who has an abscess of a maxillary sinus due to a penicillin-sensitive streptococcus, etc. There are neither quantitatively definite statistical laws to be invoked nor any rational means for the assignment of quantitatively <u>exact</u> values (believed to be true) to the logical relation "r" in such <u>typical</u> occasions in use of probabilistic inference in clinical medicine. However, recognizing that events of interest in nature may be complex, such inferences in medical explanation (or prediction) may yet be accepted in a great many contexts as adequate, in spite of their quantitative inexactness. This leads to the clinician's use of another kind of probabilities.

Objective Probabilities

As previously discussed in chapter 2, probabilities for our purposes can be approached in two general ways: objective and subjective. Frequentists use objective methods, observing numbers of events or states, preferably large numbers of such observations accumulated by long runs. It has been said that this sense of probability originated in games of chance at least as early as the seventeenth century.[43] This model has flourished in today's various games of chance, not only in casinos but popular power ball games. Interestingly, these games have similarity with Hempel's example (above) of calculating probabilities when drawing marked balls from an urn—games perhaps played centuries ago! Simple models like this are generally intuitive and relied upon. Even long run observable events used in explaining or predicting rain, for example, are sometimes relied upon. Much more complex systems, such as living organisms, are commensurably complicated and difficult for scientific explanation and prediction. This applies particularly to humans, given their minds, creativity, values, individualism, etc. In short, subjective probability is needed in medical diagnosis.[44-45]

Subjective Probability

Hempel's work surfaces once again, this time dealing with his example of an octogenarian having a weak heart and a streptococcal infection. These two joint conditions would be called "comorbidities." Would either of the two affect the other? Yes, either could do so—in fact, in this example, they may have begun as a single condition: an infection of the heart. Infection might then migrate to other sites. Many other comorbidities may be recognized at presentation or develop as complications. How common are comorbidities? They are very common, especially in older patients. Boyd[46] reviews a study by Anderson[47] thus: "In 1999, 48% of Medicare beneficiaries aged 65 years or older had at least 3 chronic medical conditions [in a set of 9] and 21% had 5 or more. Health care costs for individuals with at least 3 chronic conditions accounted for 89% of Medicare's annual budget." The complexity of such patients would increase if a larger set of chronic conditions (15) were surveyed.[48] Focusing on CPGs (Clinical Practice Guidelines), Boyd states further: "It is evident that CPGs designed by specialty-dominated committees for managing single disease, provide clinicians little guidance about caring for older patience with multiple disease."[49] Older patients are also susceptible to a myriad of non-chronic diseases. These would normally include streptococcal infection, as in our octogenarian. Unfortunately, if not successfully treated, this infection can cause a serious and at least sometimes chronic (or fatal) disease, rheumatic fever, than can potentially damage the heart, joints, and other organs. Younger patients can also have multiple diseases at once, if less likely to be chronic. Objective probabilities commonly do not offer good fit in management of one or many patients, i.e., one or many individual cases. The more complicated patients' conditions become, the more muddled and less useful objective (frequentist) probabilities tend to become, shifting the clinician to use of subjective probabilities. The clinician can then delve into her/his entire body of medical knowledge, her/his experiences and the values of the patient, etc. This in part clarifies the interest in Bayesian models, open to subjective probabilities in medical reasoning. Like the Bayesian model, to some degree, the covering law model in the diagnostic process is also open to subjective (and objective) probabilities, but wider.

Summary

In spite of the qualifications needed in the adaptation of Hempel's account of inductive-statistical explanation of individual events to the clinician's domain, the inductive-statistical model presented seems adequate in the schematic representation of the formal structure of such arguments. With the qualifications suggested, the model is therefore adopted here in relation to those probabilistic explanations (and predictions) in clinical medicine to which such a relatively statistical analysis is appropriate, i.e., where neither a deductive-nomological analysis nor its tendency-laws variant is applicable.

Before proceeding to the question of the uses of explanation and prediction in clinical diagnosis, some matters relating to our account this far will be discussed.

REFERENCES AND FOOTNOTES: CHAPTER 5

1. Hempel, C. G. "Aspects of Scientific Explanations," The Free Press, New York, 1965

2. Hempel, C. G., and Oppenheim P., "Studies in the Logic of Explanation" Philosophy of Science, 15: 135-175, 1948

3. Rosenberg, A., Op cit, pp30-36

4. Okasha S., "Philosophy of science, a very short introduction." Oxford University Press (2002), Oxford UK, ""Explanation in science" pp 40-57

5. Hempel, C., Op cit., p249

6. Steven Henry has emphasized the importance of tacit knowledge in clinical medicine, in "Recognizing Tacit Knowledge in Medical Epistemology," Theoretical Medicine and Bioethics, 26:187-213, Springer 2006. Cf also Malcom Potts' refreshing article "Controversy: Parachute approach to evidence based medicine," http://www.ncbi.nih.gov/pmc/articles/PMC1584330/ 6/26/2013

7. Rosenberg, Op cit, pp 44-45

8. Hempel, C. G., "Aspects of Scientific Explanation" Op cit, p423.

9. Scriven, M., "Truism as the Ground for Historical Explanation," in Gardiner, P.,(ed.)): Theories of History. New York: The Free Press (1959) pp 460 – 461. Contrast Scriven's discussion) of the not exactly correct Gas Laws (e.g., Van der Waal's) with the following example of a universal law from

10. Hempel, C G: "Any gas expands when heated under constant pressure." (Op. cit., p. 377).

11. Dewey, J., How We Think (Boston: D. C. Heath and Co., (1910), ch. VI.62

12. Hempel, C G, Op. cit., pp. 335-36.

13. In our example, this point would be affected by, among other things, inaccuracies in the Gas Laws. While such inaccuracies appear not to

concern Hempel in relation to this example (I think properly), they are cited by Scriven among reasons for rejecting the deductive model of explanation. The above discussion also connects with Hempel's point that explanations in science have to do with only certain <u>aspects</u> of "concrete events"; but it should additionally be noted that these "aspects" can be more or less exactly characterized. Consider, by way of a medical example, the aspect "fever" in the following imaginary but plausible dialogue:

14. Consider this dialogue:

    A: "Why does Mr. Peterson have a fever?"

    B: "He has pneumonia."

    A: "Oh. But why has his temperature remained so high all day?"

    B: "Well, he has extensive lobar consolidation, he is dehydrated, and specific treatment was only started yesterday.

    A: "I see. And why has his temperature gone up 0.1° during the past hour?"

    B: (baffled): "Who can say?"

    E.g., experienced mycologists sometimes mistakenly consume poisonous mushrooms. On the other hand, there are species that are "fool-proof" even for novices.

15. Scriven, M. , Op cit, pp443-475

16. Kuhn, T. S., "The Structure of Scientific Revolutions," 2nd ed., Chicago: Univ. of Chicago Press, 1970, p15. Kuhn comments on "… established crafts like medicine, calendar making and metallurgy."

17. Brodbeck, M. "Explanation, Prediction, and Imperfect Knowledge." in <u>Readings in the Philosophy of the Social Sciences</u>." New York. The MacMillan Co., 1968, pp375-376 Ms. Brodbeck characterizes "imperfect knowledge" thus: "any law, whether it be about physical objects, persons or societies, is 'imperfect' if it does not permit us to compute (predict or postdict) the state of the system, either an individual or a group, at <u>any</u> moment from its state at <u>one</u> moment," and says of such knowledge: "The inadequacies of such 'imperfect' knowledge do not

affect the possibility of deduction. Not only do we sometimes know enough to deduce some of the laws... but all kinds of deductions can be made from the imperfect laws themselves, whether or not they are in turn deducible from something else" (italics original). Considering the "imperfect" universal "all men are mortal" (and its deductive uses), Brodbeck observes that "... such non-quantitative universal generalizations, as well as many laws of the biological and social sciences or statistical laws generally, are not necessarily 'vague.'"

18. Statistical techniques are particularly applicable in managing the inaccuracies arising from errors of measurement.

19. Rosenberg, A. Op cit, pp 73-75

20. Quine, W. V. O., "Word and Object," 2nd ed (2013), The MIT Press, Cambridge Massachusetts, pp 229-233, 245

21. Defined with or without the aid of statistics.

22. Groopman J.; Op cit., pp243,267

23. But universals used in situations in the uncertain fringe of their scope might be included in this class, e.g., a normal vitamin B_{12} absorption one day after total gastrectomy might result from residual "intrinsic-factor" etc.

24. The terminology here is not intended to be very important. It is meant as a suggestive way of referring to those statements whose logic of use may resemble that of general causal laws, although not quite meeting the latter's standard of consistent success in their applications.

25. It is an ordinary deductive account with the assumption of the satisfaction of "C".

26. Hempel, C. G. Op cit,

27. Rosenberg, A., Op cit., pp40-44

28. Hacking I. Cambridge University Press, U.K., (First ed. 1965,), New York, Cambridge University Press, (2016) "Logic of Statistical Inference."

29. Hempel, C. G/, Op cit, p387

30. Note that in inductive reasoning even very long runs do not entirely dispel uncertainty.

31. Cramer, H., <u>Mathematical Methods of Statistics</u> (Princeton: Princeton Univ. Press, 1946), pp. 148-50.

32. Hempel, op. cit. p389

33. Hempel C., Ibid., p390

34. Hempel C, Ibid., p390

35. Hempel C., Ibid., p390

36. It seems that the former will in general contain reference to a more complete set of causal conditions, relevant to the occurrence of the event to be explained, than will the latter.

37. Hempel C.,, Op cit. , p.390

38. Hempel, ibid.,, 400-401

39. Carnap, R., "Logical Foundations of Probability" Chicago University Press (1950) p,211

40. Hempel, Op cit, p.397

41. The reason for this more stringent requirement in clinical medicine can be understood in the joint light of the important attached by the clinician to the individual case, and of our construal (in consonance with Hempel's account) of scientific explanation as answering a question "why?". While in deductive explanation an acceptable answer to such a question is generally provided by the statement of acceptable premises (including laws, etc.) from which the explanandum-statement can be inferred, the situation in respect to probabilistic explanation is more complex. In clinical medicine, at least, the statement of true statistical premises from which the explanandum-statement follows with a certain (even a high) probability, even when the premises meet the requirement of including all <u>known</u> relevant information, by no means insures their acceptability as an adequate probabilistic explanation of the event in question. Such acceptability here often requires more, viz., that an explanation be deemed the best of all feasible (within the framework of clinical knowledge) probabilistic explanations, hence

that it take into account all (or as much as can reasonably be obtained, etc.) information known (or believed, within that framework) to be of <u>potential</u> relevance to the explanandum-event. Thus, while the fact that a recovered strain of streptococcus is penicillin-resistant might provide an adequate explanation of why a culture of this micro-organism failed to show inhibition of growth in the presence of a certain concentration of penicillin, it would not be adequate without the conjunction

42. Hempel, op. cit., p. 390.

43. Hacking I., Ibid. p.10.

44. Cunningham T., Classification, disease and evidence: new essays in the philosophy of medicine Vol. 7 2015 Dordrecht; New York; Springer (2015) "Chapter: objectivity, scientificity, and the dualistic epistemology of medicine" pp1-17

45. Croskerry P. Canadian Journal Anesthesiology; 2005; 52:6 "The theory and practice of clinical decision-making"ppR1-R8

46. Boyd C. JAMA, August 10, Vol. 294 (2005) "Clinical Practice Guidelines and Quality of Care for Older Patients With Multiple Comorbid Diseases" p 716

47. Anderson G. and Horvath J., Robert Wood Johnson Foundations Partnership for Solutions; 2002 Princeton, NJ "Conditions: Case for Ongoing Care."

48. Boyd C. Ibid., p. 716

49. Boyd C., Op cit p. 720

CHAPTER 6

The Covering–Law Model: related aspects

Given that the covering law model originated a few decades ago, it has been quite thoroughly examined and discussed by philosophers of science. As with other topics relevant to medical diagnosis, this matter stretches beyond the scope of this manuscript. Nonetheless, a few questions for discussion seem appropriate at this point.

Explanation and Prediction: Structural Identity

Since scientific law statements of either universal or probabilistic form do not in general make any particular temporal reference, referring not to particular events but only to kinds of events, their uses, conjoined with singular statements, in explanation and prediction should be logically identical under the covering-law model. Construed thus, explanation and prediction in science differ only in the practical respect of whether a logically derived description of the occurrence of a particular event takes place before (prediction) or after (explanation) its actual occurrence. Originally, this was adumbrated by Hempel and Oppenheim in relation to the deductive model. Subsequently, Hempel published the (so called) "thesis of the structural identity of explanation and prediction,"[1] which given the above discussion should hold for probabilistic as well as deductive inference in covering law reasoning. Since this thesis appears to be implicit in Hempel's covering-law model, it is not surprising that critics of the model have challenged the structural-identity thesis.

The first sub-thesis

A much discussed example, which is alleged by Scriven to show the thesis' inadequacy, is presented by him as follows:

"Suppose we know that primary syphilis only leads to the tertiary condition, paresis, once in 5000 cases, but also know that paresis, when it does occur, can only be due to the spread of a prior syphilitic infection. Then we can give a causal explanation of the occurrence of paresis (E) in a particular patient as being due to his earlier condition of syphilis, although at the time of that earlier condition we would not be able to predict E-- indeed, we would confidently and rationally predict that E would not occur."[2]

But the issues involved in this example are more complex than Scriven's simplified account suggests. His claims contain factual and logical mistakes that vitiate the purported conclusion of the example.

It is useful here to distinguish two possible senses in which the word "probable" can come into play in respect to "explanation," viz., (1) in the sense already discussed in the logical relation of the explanans to the explanandum-statement, and (2) in the sense of the possible truth of the explanans. These different senses are plainly not to be confused.[3]

Suppose Scriven's example to be factually unproblematic, i.e., that the only (known) cause of paresis ("P") is syphilis ("S"), and that "S" only infrequently leads to "P" (the reported incidence of what is here meant by "paresis" among patients with untreated syphilis actually meets about 5%). On an occurrence of "P" a clinician may then infer (deduce, in the given knowledge situation) the antecedent occurrence in the patient of "S". (In diagnostic terminology, "P" represents a finding that is pathognomonic in respect to the disease "S"). What bearing does the possibility of such an inference have on the explanatory force of "S" in relation to "P" (accepting, I think properly, Scriven's claim that "S" has some explanatory force in relation to "P" given their stated relation)?

It seems to me to have no significant bearing at all. Contrast with the example the more typical diagnostic situation where a causal explanation is sought for a manifestation "M" (of which "P" is here construed as an instance), which is known to be a result of one of several possible diseases, say "A" and "B". Those two might then figure in alternative possible explanations of "M" in a given context. Now, the determination (however it may be made, say by virtue of an unshared manifestation "O") of which of these alternatives is correct does not, I think, affect the explanatory strength of the disease hypothesis selected in relation to "M". Assignment of probability (in sense {2} above) to rival diagnostic hypotheses in explanatory accounts of a given event does not alter their certain (deductive, causally complete) or probabilistic (inductive, causally incomplete) logical relations with the event; an explanation known to be correct (among possible alternatives) may be none-the-less probabilistic (in sense {1} above).

To deny the correctness or significance of this (e.g., by attending only in certain contexts to psychological and not to logical aspects of explanation) is not consistent with the varying degrees of inadequacy commonly ascribed to logically probabilistic explanations, even in situations of use where they are firmly thought to be correct. The relation of syphilis to paresis is typical in that a good deal of medical investigation has been directed at the determination of factors causally contributory to the occurrence of paresis (signs and symptoms) given syphilis, i.e., to a resolution of the residual "why?" associated with an explanatory account of paresis involving reference to syphilis. Such causally incomplete explanations as the example illustrates remain (logically) probabilistic, whatever the degree of certainty with which they may be known or believed to pertain in given instances.

As Scriven exaggerates the explanatory potency of syphilis in relation to paresis, he also exaggerates its predictive impotence. His remark that, given syphilis, "we would confidently and rationally predict that [paresis] would not occur" is distinctly misleading. Correctly stated, in a given case of untreated syphilis we would rationally assign, on the basis of the probabilities associated with their respective arguments, a considerably higher probability to the (truth of the) predictive statement that paresis will not occur than to the statement that it will occur. The non-zero probability of the latter is supported, ex-hypothesis, only by the statements asserting the occurrence of syphilis and its weak association with paresis. The uses of these predictive statements will depend of course on considerations of utility, risk, etc. It should not be supposed that the statement with the lesser probability of truth has no legitimate predictive status, or that it is logically inferior or in all contexts less important than the other. In clinical medicine, in fact, relative importance is ascribed to these predictive statements in the converse manner. For it is just the statement that paresis will occur in a given case of untreated syphilis that provides the rationale for treatment of the disease, to forestall, as far as possible, the occurrence of paresis. The more probably true statement that paresis will not occur, even in the absence of treatment, clearly does not exhaust the predictive possibilities in such a situation. Again, the psychology of prediction, as of explanation, while important and interesting in certain contexts, is not sufficient in an explication of either concept in relation to science. The false optimism implicit in Scriven's simplified sense of prediction in his discussion of this example would be quite inappropriate in clinical medicine or in other contexts.

An error in Scriven's presentation of this example should be noted. The mistake rests on a conflation of a disease with its manifestations. The distinction between these concepts is implicit in accepted explanatory usage, where a disease may explain its manifestations but usually not vice versa. While one disease may serve in an explanation of another (e.g., mucoviscidosis in relation to chronic pulmonary disease), it cannot serve in an explanation of itself. Neither, recognizing that a disease may persist in time and exhibit itself in various ways, can one manifestation of a disease as a rule serve in a causal explanation of another.[4]

Now, if the paresis of syphilis is construed as a manifestation of this disease, the constellation of signs and symptoms (weakness, tremor, dementia, etc.) that the term would generally be understood to designate is (a) highly variegated between individual cases and (b) not peculiar to syphilis.[5] On this construal not only is the occurrence of paresis only probabilistic in relation to syphilis, but the converse is also true. While these relations are common in diagnostic medicine, and while on this construal syphilis (as has been argued) may usefully serve in a probabilistic explanation of paresis, the interpretation here does not conform to the assumptions of Scriven's argument.[6]

Scriven's example therefore neither shows what he claims concerning the explanatory and predictive relations of syphilis to paresis, nor in fact to be correctly formulated. It falls short of being an effective counter-example to the contended logical symmetry of explanation and prediction in science.

The second sub-thesis

The sub-thesis that every adequate scientific prediction is potentially an explanation appears more problematic than the first. Several points are of interest.

Hempel examines the relation of "Koplik spots"[7] to other manifestations of measles as providing a possible counter-example to this sub-thesis. Suppose that Koplik spots are always followed by other manifestations of measles. A law statement of this association might then be used in deductive-nomological prediction of such later manifestations, but would be of questionable adequacy in their explanation.

Hempel considers this example indecisive on these grounds, as follows:

". . . the reluctance to regard the appearance of Koplik spots as explanatory may well reflect doubts as to whether, as a matter of universal law, those spots are always followed by the later manifestations of measles. Perhaps a local inoculation with a small amount of measles virus would produce the spots without leading to a full-blown case of the measles. If this were so, the appearance of the spots would still afford a usually reliable basis for predicting the occurrence of further symptoms, since exceptional circumstances of the kind just mentioned would be extremely rare; but the generalization that Koplik spots are always followed by later symptoms of the measles would not express a law and thus could not properly support a corresponding D-N explanation."[8]

It seems clear however that reluctance to regard Koplik spots as thus explanatory depends not on the question whether their associations with later manifestations of measles are universal or statistical, but derives rather from their theoretically accepted <u>causal irrelevance</u> (as <u>spots</u>) in relation to such other manifestations. Moreover, Hempel's argument does not attend to the possible force of the example in relation to the symmetry questions of corresponding probabilistic explanations and predictions, if the associations of interest are indeed only statistical.

A more satisfactory analysis of this example, and its weakness as a putative counter-example to the <u>second</u> sub-thesis, again depends on a recognition of the distinction between a disease and its manifestations, and on an examination of "Koplik spots" in relation to this distinction.

Construed as a mere <u>manifestation</u> of disease, Koplik spots are not, certainly not always, distinctive. They must be distinguished from other lesions of the oral mucosa having a more-or-less similar appearance (e.g., thrush, aphthous stomatitis, small traumatic dental ulcers, submucous fat, inspissated mucus, etc.). This differentiation involves theoretic judgements ordinarily requiring consideration of such various other factors as the patient's age, history (including possible disease exposure and immunity), presence or absence of other signs and symptoms, laboratory results, etc. Far from being a nosologically neutral descriptive predicate, Koplik spots in fact ascribes to a patient not only a certain kind of disease manifestation, but also the specific etiology (measles) of this manifestation. For whatever their appearance, oral lesions of any other etiology are not (in accepted usage) Koplik spots. Like dementia paralytica, the term is etiologically defined.

While there is a well-accepted association between Koplik spots, so understood, and other manifestations of measles, there is no accepted association between such other manifestations and

Koplik-like spots. Only the tacit reference to <u>measles</u> in the anteced-ent of the stated association provides the basis for its scientific use in prediction of the later manifestations of this disease—but the same reference would also provide a basis for its use in their explanation.[9]

These purported counter-examples to the <u>second</u> sub-thesis have a common form, in which a cause "C" is <u>known</u> (or theoretically accepted) to be associated with two or more effects, e.g., "E" and "E'", one of which (say E) typically precedes the other. The claim is then made that an occurrence of E <u>itself</u> supports a predictive inference to E', but is on the other hand—given the assumed causal knowledge—not adequate in the explanation of E'. However, the first part of this claim, on which the force of the examples hinges, seems specious. For the scientific acceptability of the predictive inference to E', under the stated conditions, is wholly dependent on the (tacitly or openly) asserted occurrence of C, and the integrity in a given context of its causal relation with E'. This dependence is most clear in situations where E is further known to be a possible effect of various different causes (having other effects which may or may not include E'), or where the causal link between C and E' may be altered or breached by the influence of other factors. Situations of both kinds are abundant in clinical medicine, for example the fever and rash of measles, and the effects on either or both of the administration of hyper-immune serum. In such cases a judgement on the occurrence of C, and other potentially relevant factors, typically becomes explicit. That the same kind of judgement may in some contexts be only implicit does not lessen its importance in such inferences. The inadequacy of constru-ing a predictive argument of elliptical form (e.g., from E to E') in narrowly <u>prima facie</u> terms is quite apparent in contexts where the prediction concerned is of some actual <u>consequence</u>, for example in clinical medicine where practical neglect of known pertinent causal considerations could be plainly remiss. Equally unsatisfactory, in my view, would be a similar neglect of causal knowledge in the assessment of such predictions, in particular the role of boundary and antecedent conditions, and importantly unexpected intrusive conditions able to steer the prediction awry. This is a matter of empirical error, not a logical flaw in the symmetry sub-thesis. For example:

A Thought Experiment – two bakers

Two proud bakers often compete, but on one occasion baker 1 showed up a few hours before baker 2. By the time the latter arrived, baker 1 was ready to show her/him a freshly baked cake. As the cake was particularly beautiful and delicious, baker 1 explained in detail the recipe (including several time tested generalizations). Baker 2 went to work, predicting that her/his cake would be just as delightful as the first. Unfortunately, however, the second cake turned out flat, and not so delicious. Soon enough, baker 2 remembered she/he had mistakenly inverted the ratio of baking soda (sodium bicarbonate, a chemical base) and baking powder (a smaller amount of sodium bicarbonate mixed with an acidic ingredient), the latter having significantly less strength in leavening. If readable and not confusing, should the recipe be seen as faulty?

Empirical generalizations

Hempel asserts, "A scientific prediction may be based on a finite set of data which includes no laws and which would have no explanatory force." However, ... "if this event actually occurs, the test data clearly do not provide an explanation for it."[10]

Such a situation might lead to potentially useful connections, though. All sets of scientific data are finite, and Hempel provides no compelling reason for believing the hypotheses here considered not to be general claims. Neither is any reason suggested for believing the associations expressed not to be of a causal nature (unlike the association of E with E', above). Indeed, the contrary would ordinarily be supposed. As general causal hypothesis, the stated associations would seem to provide a <u>logical</u> footing for exploring explanation as for prediction.

It cannot be important in this that the details of the causal relationships involved are not known, for there are many examples of acceptable explanation in which this is the case, and in no case can such details be known to have been fully elucidated. Neither can it be important here that the instances of an empirical regularity (as in the examples) provide no explanation for it, for this of course never occurs. Nor can the explanatory function of a generalization asserting such a regularity depend on its own explanation (i.e., derivation from other laws). Such a requirement would be consistent neither with common usage nor with the covering-law model itself, for there will always be some higher-order that which are not so derivable.

Practically, if a certain chemical is known to inhibit the growth of cancer cells, or if an increase in the temperature of an electrical conductor is known to be accompanied by an increase in its electrical resistance, statements of these associations must surely have explanation as well as predictive usefulness in relation to particular instances of such phenomena.

These examples, like those discussed above, seem not conclusive as counter-examples to either sub-thesis.

Explanation by Concept

An interesting proposal of a possible mode of explanation in history has been proposed by Dray, a Canadian philosopher of history in the twentieth century. Calling it "explanation by concept," Dray suggests this is an alternative kind of explanation in science, where the explanation is deemed to answer an interrogative "What?" rather than "Why?"[11] This proposal is of interest especially in relation to syndrome concepts, and their explanatory role in clinical medicine.

Discussing changes which took place in late eighteenth century England, Dray quotes from Muir[12] the remark, "It was not merely an economic change that was thus beginning; it was a social revolution,"[13] observing that "the historian here makes no attempt to tell us either why or how the events under investigation came about. Yet the assertion, 'It was a social revolution,' is an explanation nonetheless. It explains what happened as a social revolution,"[14] and that "the explanation is given by finding a satisfactory classification of what seems to require explanation."[15] Insofar as any generalization is needed for the kind of explanation envisaged, its form and use are elucidated by Dray as follows: "For what is to be explained is a collection of happenings or conditions x, y, and z; and the relevant generalization would be of the form: 'X, y and z amount to a Q'. Such an explanatory generalization is summative; it allows us to refer to x, y and z collectively as 'a so-and-so'. And historians find it intellectually satisfying to be able to represent the events and conditions they study as related in this way."[16]

Thus, the thrust of Dray's proposal, centered on certain empiric phenomena to be explained, e.g., x, y, and z, are not to be regarded as manifestations of a causal phenomenon Q, but rather as its definitional constituents. Like the image in a jigsaw puzzle, Q does not itself exist before its parts are in place. On this interpretation, analogous examples can be found among medical syndromes, different from etiologically classified diseases (e.g., measles, a specific virus infection of which subclinical cases—with minimal manifestations—may be diagnosed). While some syndromes have been treated as diagnoses, many have been thoroughly investigated, revealing previously unknown abnormalities causing manifestations of the syndrome (e.g., Cushing's syndrome, Reiter's syndrome, etc.), leading to new causal knowledge used in diagnosis and treatment of underlying diseases.

A prominent feature of syndromes is a tendency to cluster their manifestations in more or less typical patterns. These patterns can be helpful for the clinician to bring to mind potential diagnoses. Such patterns however are quite variable, and in general simply manifestations—signs and symptoms. Thus, after her/his new patient history and physical examination the clinician will start a "work-up" (testing) in the diagnostic process. Patients exhibiting pattern recognition are managed similarly in this process. There are some exceptions; for example, an otherwise healthy patient with a small skin laceration, with no other complaints, may simply have appropriate surgery.

Historical studies of social and political revolutions, or other significant societal shifts, may use concept explanation to help glean new knowledge or insight in such phenomena. A sort of summative classification, focused only on empiric manifestations, this model is blind to causal associations. It will not be adopted here.

Mathematical Models of Explanation

Alex Rosenberg discusses two other counterexamples, the first proposed by Sylvan Bromberger,[17] to test the deductive-nomological (D-N) model of scientific explanation. The example goes thus: A flagpole is too high to be measured directly, so curious folks tried another approach. On a certain time on a certain day, the sunlight meets the ground at the angle of 45 degrees at the flagpole, which stands straight upright. Knowing principles of geometry, the curious and innovative folks measured the flagpole's shadow, and then calculate the height of the flagpole (50 ft.).

For some philosophers, the issue here seems to satisfy the canons of D-N explanation, but not its _pragmatics_. Referring to the flagpole, Rosenberg writes on this view as "the shadow it casts, not its cause— the desires of the Missoula city mothers to have a flagpole one foot taller than the 49-foot flagpole at Helena, Montana."[18-20] Given this, perhaps both senses of "explanation" are satisfied among others, e.g., scientists and philosophers.

On mathematical models, it should be noted that such equations from physical sciences have an important role in clinical medicine. Some have been used in clinical medicine for several decades. Prominent among these formulas include the ideal gas law, $PV = nRT$, useful in measurements of capacity and function of the respiratory system, and the Henderson–Hasselbalch equation, $pH = pKa + \log^{10} \{ (A\text{-})/\{HA) \}$, highly useful in managing electrolyte (acid–base) balance in body fluids. More recently other mathematical formulae have been extremely useful in medical imaging (e.g., photons/gamma rays, sound waves/"echo," positrons/charged light anti-matter particles, and MRI/oscillating magnetic fields), and in radiation therapy (e.g., photons/gamma rays, electrons/charged light particles, and protons/charged heavy particles). It would be fair to say that new knowledge of this kind provides numerous game changers in modern medical science. Importantly, clinicians weave new knowledge into their reasoning, both within the diagnostic process and the management of their patients. In fact, they are mandated to do so.

Some critics may view clinical science as standing on the legs of basic science, a view that is not new. Thomas Kuhn (American, 1922-1996), in his book _The Structure of Scientific Revolutions_, alluded to "established crafts like medicine, calendar making and metallurgy."[21]

Kuhn was a physicist, and was mistaken about medicine. Medicine is not an "established craft," it is a dynamic science. Like many other sciences, it is true that medical science draws in part on physics (and chemistry, etc.), whereas most physicists would agree that the opposite is not true. As a research fellow in physical chemistry (some time ago), I recognized the importance of an admixture of physics, but there seemed minimal (or none) vice-versa. Would this signal a trend leading to lots of thin knowledge among "basic scientists" of very complex human sciences? Be that as it may, but with emphasis of the scope and depth of complexity in medical science, including elements of basic sciences and much more. This issue will be discussed further in a later chapter. For now, the claim is simply that mathematical formulae fit and are useful in clinical medicine.

Law-Testing in Clinical Medicine

Returning briefly to an earlier topic, and recalling discussion of the deductive-nomological schema, the covering-law model of explanation and prediction is also important to investigative aspects of clinical medicine in sharing a logical nexus with medical diagnosis.

In terms of this model, the non-occurrence of an event "e" whose description is inferred from statements of initial and boundary conditions and universal generalizations only logically implies the falsity of one of these premises. It is claimed that such situations are common in diagnostic contexts, and that when confronted with these circumstances clinicians are free to scrutinize and select between the relevant premises, rejecting that which they believe most likely to be false. Diagnostic testing challenges, then, not only particular diagnostic propositions (although these are usually of most immediate concern), but also the law-statements with which such propositions are conjoined in clinical inference.

It has been argued that many such law-statements are distinctly clinical, and are not amenable to testing in other contexts. As in other sciences, moreover, there is in clinical medicine a frequent introduction of new (and revision of old) general hypotheses. Given this situation and the accepted goals of clinical medicine, it is not surprising or unreasonable that many clinicians should regard the critical <u>evaluation</u> of such law-statements, variously accepted as premises in clinical arguments, not only as an option but also as an important responsibility. For theirs is the ultimate responsibility in their use.

It has long been recognized that natural laws in science can never be verified. Accepted laws are accepted only tentatively, and are always subject to revision or rejection. Such changes are most characteristic of a science in rapid development, as is now the case in medicine.

Few, I think, would deny the importance of medical knowledge or of its ongoing process of appraisal and development. It has been argued that clinicians are in a uniquely favorable position to put such knowledge to the test. These considerations strongly discredit the view that medical diagnosis in general either can or should be reduced to rote or recipe as would be required for diagnosis by computer or technician.[22] The view taken here is rather that of the clinician who interprets data in the light of available knowledge, and who tests her/his knowledge along with particular diagnostic suppositions in respect to individual cases. Case diagnosis and the testing (and development) of medical knowledge are seen as logically interwoven activities within clinical medicine. As discussed, medical knowledge is infused with theories, generally supported but with various views. A more direct and detailed explanation of the workings of the diagnostic process on this view will be taken up in the next chapter.

Summary

Consideration has been given in this chapter to the basic elements of a <u>hypotheses-inferential</u> model of the diagnostic process in clinical

Lee A Forstrom

medicine. Included in discussion were the structure and functions of diagnostic propositions, with particular attention to their explanatory role. The nature of this role has been examined in relation to the major schemas of the covering-law model of scientific explanation, exhibiting its requirement for the use of general claims or scientific law-statements. Various kinds of law-statements commonly used in clinical inference were discussed.

In spite of criticisms, a number of which were discussed, the covering-law model stands as a satisfactory (the best) means for an explication of the logic of clinical explanation and prediction. Clarifying the structure and conceptual constituents of these activities, this model also illuminates the close relation between clinical diagnosis and clinical investigation.

A more direct and detailed explanation of the workings of the diagnostic process on this view will be taken up in the next chapter.

REFERENCES AND FOOTNOTES: CHAPTER 6

1. Hempel C., op cit, pp.366-367

2. Scriven, "M. The Temporal Asymmetry of Explanation and Prediction," in Baumrin, op. cit., p. 99.

3. Sense (2) is closely connected with the "acceptability" of an explanation, i.e., to what extent it is taken to correctly identify the reasons (in science, generally, "causes") for the occurrence of the explanandum-event. In the case of a deductive explanation, the question of its acceptability is ordinarily settled by a determination of the truth of its premises (given the validity of the argument). The situation in respect to "inductive" explanation is again more complex. While no probabilistic explanation explicitly states causally sufficient conditions for the occurrence of the explanandum event, such explanations are of course only variously imperfect in this respect. The requirement that an acceptable explanation of important phenomena be the best (construing "the reasons" for an event as "all the important identifiable reasons") generates the more stringent evidential requirement for the "adequacy" of probabilistic explanations in clinical medicine, as previously discussed.

4. There are certainly many exceptions to this rule, depending on particular causal mechanisms involved. For example, congestive heart failure and tachypnea may be separate or joint "manifestations" of myocardial infarction, and the former may or may not in individual cases contribute in a causal explanation of the latter.

5. Knudsen R P, emedicine.medscape.com/article/1169231, (11/23/2016) "Neurosyphilis: Overview of Syphilis of the CNS" pp 1-3.

6. An interpretation of "paresis" which prima facie conforms (superficially) to the requirements of Scriven's argument is its construal as a condition which "results" only from syphilis as a matter not of empirical fact but of definition; i.e., "chronic syphilitic meningo-encephalitis."

This condition whose predication attributes to an individual not only a set of manifestations but also their syphilitic cause. In relation to an occurrence of dementia paralytica, therefore, "syphilis" is explanatorily redundant.

7. Small spots on the oral mucosa occurring with measles, named after H. Koplik, U. S. pediatrician (1858-1927). Cf. Tierney L M, NEJM (2006) 354:740 "Koplik Spots"/ February 16, 2006/ DOI: 10.1056/NEJMicm050576

8. Hempel, C. op cit, p375 Cf. also the following remarks by Hempel: "A condition that is nomically necessary for the occurrence of an event does not, in general, explain it; or else we would be able to explain a man's winning the first prize in the Irish sweepstakes by pointing out that he had previously bought a ticket, and that only a person who owns a ticket can win the first prize" (pp.369-70). But the statement of a nomically necessary condition can <u>sometimes</u> provide the ground for an "adequate" probabilistic explanation, for a probabilistic explanation never explicitly offers more (i.e., nomically sufficient conditions), and may offer less (as in medical explanation of a manifestation in terms of one of several possible causes). Moreover, the considerable differences between Hempel's and Scriven's examples are obviously, both in respect to the degrees of probability involved (suppose only two or three sweepstakes tickets were sold), and in the sense of "cause" relevant to the suggested explanations.

9. An explanation referring directly to measles would be more satisfactory because less ambiguous (given the way in which "Koplik spots" straddles the disease: manifestation distinction). But the above suggestion is not merely fanciful. Consider for example, the following (plausible) clinical dialogue (where clinician "A" may be seen as the verbally more fastidious and "B" as the logically subtler):

A: "Why does the Jones boy have a fever and rash this morning?"
B: "He had Koplik spots yesterday."
A: "I see. You mean because he has measles."

B: "Yes, that's what I meant."

Now consider the implausibility of a dialogue like this except for the substitution of another descriptive predicate (not involving reference to measles) for "Koplik spots."

10. Hempel, C., Op cit., p375.

11. Dray, W., "'Explaining What' in History," in Gardiner, The Free Press, Glencoe, Illinois (1959) Theories of History, pp. 403-408

12. Muir, R. A Short History of the British Commonwealth, 6th ed., (London: George Philip and Son, 1937), II, p. 123.

13. Dray, op. cit., p. 403

14. Dray, Ibid.p. 403

15. Dray, Ibid., p. 404

16. Dray, Ibid, p.406

17. Rosenberg, A., Op. cit., pp 30, 38

18. Rosenberg, A., Ibid. p.38

19. Rosenberg A., Ibid. Rosenberg offers a version of Hempel's original statements in D-N as follows: " (1) The explanation must be a valid deductive argument. (2) The explanans must contain at least one general law actually needed in the deduction. (3) The explanans must be empirically testable. (4) The sentences in the explanans must be true." pp30-31

20. Rosenberg, A. Ibid., p39

21. Kuhn, T., Univ. of Chicago Press (2nd edition, 1970) "The Structure of Scientific Revolution" p.15

22. Groopman, J., Op cit., p5

CHAPTER 7

The Diagnostic Process in the Hypotheses-Inferential Model

Introduction

In this chapter, the structure of clinical diagnosis will be more explicitly examined and characterized in terms of a hypotheses-inferential model, in the light of what has already been set forth. A simplified diagnostic situation will be discussed, followed by consideration of certain typical complexities in the more general situation. The present account will be further explored in a comparison with the statistical view.

In this discussion, I will omit further consideration of those relatively simple diseases whose definitions exhaust the evidence of abnormality (e.g., laceration of the arm), and whose logic of diagnosis is quite straightforward. To a certain extent, medical syndromes and their diagnosis share in this simplicity, but it should be recalled that the features of most syndromes are also possible effects of other (more etiologically defined) diseases. As was said earlier, a clinician must therefore ordinarily reason causally, relating evidence to various disease possibilities, even in the selection of a syndrome diagnosis. When a syndrome is not obvious (like laceration of the arm; cf., perhaps, classic cases of certain syndromes), then its logic of diagnosis will conform generally with that of other diseases (or conditions) as in the following account. Such diagnoses will therefore not receive further separate consideration.

The Clinical Diagnostic Process

Suppose a clinician is presented with a new patient. The patient's history (including her/his complaints) and physical examination (including any preliminary laboratory results) constitute the clinician's initial data, forming the basis for a certain diagnostic development. What is the nature of the process by which the clinician proceeds from this basis in the making of a diagnosis?

The answer to this question has been summed up in a passage from R. C. Cabot, cited earlier, in which the clinician's diagnostic activity is seen as that of "forming reasonable hypotheses about a case of disease and then. . . testing these hypotheses by such experiments as shall establish the correct and nullify the incorrect."[1] Numerous observers have since been influenced by this analysis as important in understanding the clinician's reasoning and actions in medical diagnosis.[2-6] Most (or all) of this literature, however, terms and deals with hypothesis-deductive models, obscuring the roles of other kinds of logic (induction and probabilistic), and over-simplifying the complexity of clinical reasoning.

Two components of this activity are distinguished. Restated, these are the formulation of a set of alternative diagnostic hypotheses, and the selection from among these of the correct diagnosis. They will be considered in turn. The assumption will first be made that there is a single correct diagnostic hypothesis—which may, however, be composite—in relation to the evidence of disease of concern in a given case.

The Selection of Diagnostic Hypotheses

As has been pointed out, most signs and symptoms of a disease are non-specified (not unique to it), being rather possible results of a more or less large number of different diseases. Given the initial evidence, therefore, the clinician must as a rule consider at least several diseases as diagnostic possibilities, as Cabot saw: "Each case should lead us to arrange before the mind's eye a selected group of reasonably probable causes for the symptoms complained of and for the signs discovered."[7] This is particularly germane to the early stages of the diagnostic process, in which the clinician compiles the well-known list of differential diagnoses. In general, the wider the class of diagnostic possibilities listed, the more likely it is to contain the correct one. The correct diagnosis may of course be added to the list at any time, but it is an important truism that the making of a diagnosis (the correct one being of cardinal interest) requires that it must first be considered.

How a clinician brings to mind sometimes called "abduction" (advocated by C. S. Peirce),[8] certain diagnostic possibilities in a given case is at least in part a matter of (psychological) conjecture. The importance in this of what is known as "pattern recognition" is often emphasized. The evidence may contain or consist of a pattern of findings so typical of (the manifestations of) a certain disease that the clinician promptly recognizes that disease as a diagnostic possibility to be distinguished from his recognizing the disease (as discussed below). Also relevant in this must be the clinician's rough knowledge of disease incidences.[9] However, the importance of this should not be greatly emphasized; uncommon diseases are also diagnosed and must be considered.

Of more interest are the grounds on which the clinician selects from those diagnostic possibilities entertained, however cursorily, in compiling his initial list of differential diagnoses. Again relevant must be her/his rough knowledge of disease incidence, but the importance of this should once more not be overstated, for uncommon (even rare) diseases are commonly included as possibilities in such lists. Of perhaps more importance is the clinician's assessment of the relative seriousness (always partly context-dependent) of a disease possibility in determining the extent of its consideration. Such things as the clinician's personal interests and familiarities must be allowed an understandable part in this. Of most interest here are two conditions I believe to be of decisive logical (and the greatest practical) importance in deciding which diagnostic possibilities should be included in a given set of differential diagnoses. Inasmuch as any such set is continually open to revision, these conditions will be recognized to obtain throughout the diagnostic process.

First condition

The first of these is suggested by Cabot's reference to diseases imagined as possible "causes of the symptoms complained of and for the signs discovered."[10] To be considered a serious possibility, then, a particular diagnostic "h_d" must be acceptable as potentially explanatory, in conjunction with known causal associations in relation to a certain body of evidence, "E^*." This will be understood to enlarge as evidence accumulates. On our assumption of a single correct diagnostic hypothesis, E^* will be at least partly similar for all rival diagnostic hypotheses, but need not include all the available evidence of disease, as some of this may already have been known to be related to disease previously diagnosed.

Second condition

The second condition is that there should be no evidence (e.g., outside E*; it will most often be a normal finding) with which the diagnostic hypothesis "h_d" is, in respect to available knowledge and theory, seen as highly incompatible. Such evidence may be diverse in type, including the known presence (or absence) of other diseases or conditions.

Suppose a clinician's knowledge situation in a given diagnostic context, including information then available to her/him about the patient, assumptions, and the medical laws and generalizations she/ he accepts, to be represented by (the class of statements) "K". Given the sense of "explain" adopted and developed above (including its probabilistic sense), the conditions for her/his acceptance in that situation of a contending diagnostic hypothesis, "h_d", as worthy of further consideration, can be put briefly as follows:

(1)   When conjoined with "K", "h_d" must provide a potential explanation of the evidence of disease, E*, for which it is held accountable.[11]

(2)   The assumption of "h_d" must be seen as compatible with "K."

That the list of differential diagnoses, as first formulated by the clinician, should be practically brief and yet include the correct hypothesis is not a small demand. For prior to the selective acquisition and use of information obtained during her/his preliminary examination, of course, a great many diseases would have to be supposed reasonably probable (or improbable). The framing of an ordinary list of differential diagnoses then requires a substantial reduction in the number of diseases to be considered, most such possibilities having already been, at least tentatively, eliminated. This process of elimination is in the early phases of diagnosis effected largely by means of condition (1), in which initial evidence draws attention to a certain class of disease possibilities. As the diagnostic process, of which the clinician's initial examination forms a beginning in continuity with the rest, proceeds, the balance of usefulness of these conditions often moves in the direction of (2). This comes about because of the relative non-specificity of most disease manifestations, and through the importance of (2) in the selective body of "K". This development will be pursued in the next section.

The Selection of a Diagnosis

A Simplified Case

Suppose in a given case that based on her/his initial information the clinician has formulated a list of differential diagnoses. Assume for now that this list contains the correct diagnosis.[12] Although such a list typically includes several diagnostic possibilities, it will be further assumed here to contain only two. Let these be called "h_a" and "h_b", and suppose that "h_a" is correct. How does the clinician arrive—or attempt to arrive—at this diagnosis?

Assuming that the diagnostic process eventually terminates in the selection of a particular diagnosis, it may first be asked, what are the general conditions whose satisfaction is commonly held to be needed in such a determination? Under what conditions, that is, is the clinician ordinarily content to accept, and act on, a diagnosis as the correct one? Although general conditions for such acceptance cannot be exactly specified, it should be clear that the clinician will not as a rule settle on a diagnosis until she/he believes it to be much—depending on context including human values/utilities—more probable, on the basis of her/his available knowledge, than its leading rivals.[13]

Second, she/he will ordinarily require that to be acceptable, any diagnosis will need to be based on an appropriately thorough evaluation, for example that her/his available knowledge at the time of its determination should be reasonably complete in respect to information seen as potentially relevant to the alternative diagnoses considered (e.g., bacteriological studies in the suspicion of infection).[14] This method cannot in my view be accurately portrayed or adequately understood as one depending on a random or prescribed sequence of information collection and analysis, a mechanical accumulation of data that the clinician at some specified time (or times) inserts into a set of formulae in calculating diagnostic probabilities. More scientific, intuitive, and personal than this, as I see it, the clinician's method involves rather a process of educated testing of alternative diagnostic hypotheses. In dealing with individual cases this process can best be understood in relation to the hypothetico-inferential model of diagnosis, which best fits traditional clinical reasoning.

Given the framework of ideas developed above, in particular those relating to clinical explanation and prediction, the central theme in this model can be briefly stated. As the conjunction of each diagnostic proposition with the clinician's information, assumptions and theory will serve in the (deductive or probabilistic) explanation of the already observed manifestations of disease, "E*", the same conjunctions will serve in the (deductive or probabilistic) predictions of other events. These predictions, formulated in accordance with the clinician's knowledge at a given time, and depending on his understanding of causal associations in health and various diseases, may relate to a wide spectrum of phenomena, including signs and symptoms and the results of a variety of laboratory, radiologic, and special procedures.

The clinician's step-wise testing of such predictions, by their comparison with selectively acquired new information, may be seen in an obvious way to confirm or disconfirm the particular diagnostic hypotheses used in their inference.

As Cabot recognized in his remark that the clinician proceeds by "testing these [diagnostic] hypotheses by such experiments as shall establish the correct and nullify the incorrect" there are, then, two major aspects, or approaches, in the method of diagnostic testing. In terms of our example and the present analysis, the clinician will select "h_a" only when she/he believes it to be much more, or sufficiently more, depending on contextual factors like those mentioned, probable than "h_b", after an appropriately thorough evaluation achieved by a process of testing these hypotheses in relation to their predictive consequences. On our assumptions, the results of such testing should increase the clinician's preference for "h_a" by, on balance, either (1) confirming "h_a" or (2) disconfirming "h_b" (or both). The relations and manner of use of these complimentary aspects of diagnostic method will be explored.

Diagnosis by "establishing" (confirming) the correct.

On the assumption that "h_a" is correct, all of its deductive predictions should succeed (assuming the truth of "K" and neglecting possible experimental error)[15] and some of its probabilistic predictions (probably) will also. When, if ever, can such successes be justifiably taken to establish the correctness of "h_a"? Clearly, this can be so only under certain special conditions.

Suppose, for example, that "h_a" successfully predicts[16] an event "e" that is not specific for the designated disease "A" (it is known to have other causes) but which is not predicted (deductively or probabilistically) by "h_b". Such an occurrence does not automatically justify the selection of "h_a" for to say that "h_b" does not predict "e" is not to say that it predicts "not-e" (a matter which will be taken up below). The occurrence of "e" might be explained, for example, in relation to some pre-existing disease—the evidence of "e" might be part of "E" but not "E*." The effect of "e" on the clinician's decision between "h_a" and "h_b" will then be determined by her/his evaluation of its occurrence, including its temporal relations with other events, in the light of her/his understanding of its causal relations with all other diseases or conditions present or considered. Even when evidence of its occurrence is accepted as within "E*," for which an explanation is sought in terms of some member of the accepted set of differential diagnoses, it could be taken to establish "h_a" (through elimination of "h_b" by condition (I) above) only on the strength of the assumptions that this list in fact contains the correct diagnosis, and that "e" is in fact never (or almost never) an effect of disease "B." Given a degree of uncertainty on both these counts, the clinician would not routinely accept "h_a" straight away in such a situation, but would continue the diagnostic testing.

Suppose, however, that "e" is regarded as specific for "A" (i.e., it is not known to have any other causes). In such circumstances, an occurrence of "e" (in clinical parlance a "pathognomonic" finding) might be taken to establish the presence of "A".

However, there is clearly a flaw in this: to say that "A" is the only known cause of "e" is not to say that "A" is known (or can be known) to be the only cause of "e", as the latter may always be found to have other causes, among diseases newly or previously recognized. Far from being exceptional, this development has in fact proved to be the rule for many such findings.

"Pectoriloquy," for example, was once seen as pathognomonic for "pulmonary phthisis" (no longer an accepted disease entity); it is now recognized as a sign of various other diseases.[17] The mistaken belief that a positive Wasserman reaction was specific for syphilis led to the erroneous treatment with arsenical compounds of numerous patients without this disease. Renal papillary necrosis, once thought fairly specific for diabetes mellitus (but occurring also with severe pyelonephritis and obstruction), has been recognized among patients with analgesic abuse. The physical finding of cogwheel respiration, once considered pathognomonic for pulmonary tuberculosis, is now regarded as non-specific, etc.

Given this experience, it is not surprising that most clinicians are wary of accepting any individual finding as establishing the presence of a particular disease. Relatively few disease manifestations are now regarded as pathognomonic.[17] It should be observed, moreover, that the occurrence of such a manifestation may be only more or less probable in relation to instances of the disease with which it is known to be associated; the disease may often be present without it. In spite of their special interest and appeal, then, the use of pathognomonic individual findings is of limited general importance in clinical diagnosis.

It is possible, on the other hand, that certain combinations of findings (e.g., "$e_1, e_2, \ldots e_n$") might be highly specific for particular diseases. Such combinations and their uses have been pursued especially by those researchers concerned with diagnosis by statistical methods. However, the general importance of such findings in diagnosis is subject to the same kinds of limitation as that of individual pathognomonic findings. Not many combinations of disease manifestations are regarded as specific for a given disease, and a combination regarded as even relatively specific for such a disease may only sometimes accompany its presence. Indeed, what is gained in such combinations on the one hand tends to be lost on the other. For the probability of occurrence of some such set of features—"$e_1, e_2, \ldots e_n$"—in an instance of the disease cannot be greater than, and will ordinarily be less than, the probability of occurrence of its least probable member. Inasmuch as several members of the set may be probabilistic in relation to the disease, the frequency of their joint occurrence among such patients will often (depending on their various degrees of statistical independence) be quite low. In general the more additions that are made to the set "e_1, e_2, ... e_n" to increase its specificity for a given disease, the less sensitive it will tend to be (assuming some degree of statistical independence between its members) as a test for the presence of the disease. Few such formulations of specific combinations of findings would therefore be accepted as expressing necessary conditions for the diagnosis of particular diseases. Neither, in fact, would many find general acceptance among clinicians as providing sufficient conditions for the same purposes; in too many situations some other disease or diseases would require consideration.[18] Moreover, the clinician must not cherry pick, but rather gather all relevant and available evidence for use in her/his diagnostic pursuit.

A related approach held in the view that diagnoses may sometimes be established by pattern recognition. Given that certain diseases may exhibit general patterns of manifestations, it is held that the evidence may in some cases be so typical of the manifestations of a particular disease that the clinician immediately recognizes its presence. For example, acromegaly and hyperthyroidism patients commonly present with such salient manifestations as to quickly bring the disease to the clinician's mind. In past times that might have been the entire diagnosis, whereas today the diseases are likely to be further tested to refine the diagnoses. For example, hyperthyroidism can stem from several sources (e.g., Grave's disease, Plummer's disease, hot nodule, various drugs, etc.). These conditions belong in differing causal chains and require different therapies.

It is no doubt true that the selection of a diagnosis is commonly affected by such recognition. However, while pattern recognition may be important in suggesting (bringing to mind) for the clinician the possible presence of a disease, perhaps in influencing her/his diagnostic preference—"it just looks like a case of 'A'—it is not often a sufficient method for determining a diagnosis. Few clinicians would now be willing to accept unchallenged the diagnosis of any serious illness on this basis alone. The importance of such recognition in diagnosis, moreover, would seem prominent only in relation to cases of disease presenting in highly typical or classic form, usually in a full-blown stage of development. Even in such relatively infrequent cases, most clinicians would test a diagnosis with a thoroughness appropriate to its prognostic and therapeutic implications, together with alternative possibilities, before accepting it as established.[19,-20]

Diagnosis by pattern recognition, then, like other techniques centering on the use of information seen as directly confirmatory for particular diagnoses, is rarely sufficient in the selection of a diagnosis. Neither is the usefulness of those objectively described features that are regarded as relatively specific for certain diseases to be minimized. Such features tend to differentiate certain classes of disease (e.g., those that can result in chest pain, anemia, abnormal serum enzymes, etc.), working thereby to suggest particular diagnostic hypotheses, but they also work in the elimination of others. The appraisal of such features in terms only of their directly confirmatory value for given diagnostic hypotheses does not provide an adequately general account of their use, or that of other kinds of information in clinical diagnostic method. Such an account must include a second aspect in this method, as suggested by Cabot, that of "nullifying the incorrect."

Diagnosis by "nullifying" (disconfirming) the incorrect.

It has been argued that there are few manifestations of disease recognized in clinical medicine as genuinely specific (pathognomonic) for particular diseases, and that formally designed combinations of manifestations for use in the same way (specific, unless by fiat) are in general neither wholly specific nor in the frequency of their potential occasions of use being adequate as indicators for the presence of particular diseases. Fortunately, clinicians are not bound to the use of such specific diagnostic criteria.

Consider again our hypothetical example. Suppose now that in this particular case the process of testing reveals not one but several findings predicted (and at least partly therefore looked for) by "h_a" but not (based on available knowledge) predicted by "h_b". Given that any one such finding might not—and probably would not—end the diagnostic process by deciding in favor of "h_a", several such outcomes might well do so. Whether or not such new evidence—assumed to lie within E*; the clinician's interpretation of this will again depend on the context—would finally result in the selection of "h_a", it should by condition (I) finally result in the rejection of "h_b." This would clearly be a useful outcome.

It should be apparent, however, that there is another route, more direct and potentially more effective, to the same result, by the testing of what "h_b" does predict. Now, on the supposition that diseases "A" and "B" have some kinds of manifestations in common, including, ex hypothesi essentially all of those described in the initial evidence E*, it may be expected that a certain number of the predictions of "h_b" will succeed. Given that this diagnosis is incorrect, many of its predictions should fail. In particular, those predictions of "h_b" may be expected to fail in relation to evidence incorporated into E*, not

147

otherwise explained, which are not also predictions of "h_b". Such failures, seen as disconfirmatory for "h_b", will clearly work to increase the clinician's preference for "h_a" as the relatively more probable of the two diagnoses. The extent to which this occurs will depend on the nature of the failed predictions. These may be of two main types.

"Strict" Predictions

These must be based on the use of ordinary causal laws or statements of invariable association. If "h_b" can be fitted to any of these law-statements, the failure of one of its deductively inferable predictions (particularly if repeatable) will ordinarily result in rejection of "h_b," by incorporation into "E^*" and hence into "K" of evidence incompatible with its assumption (condition (2)). Thus, following examples discussed earlier, and given specifiable conditions, a normal hemoglobin electrophoresis would result in most clinician's rejection of a diagnosis of sickle-cell disease; a normal glucose-tolerance test in the rejection of diabetes mellitus; a normal spinal-fluid analysis in the rejection of dementia paralytica; etc.

Of course, pertinent specifiable conditions are not always satisfied to permit the use of test results in the above manner. Such results are always evaluated in individual cases in relation to the clinician's knowledge and assessment of causally relevant factors. However, the failure of a prediction considered strict in relation to a given knowledge situation is commonly taken without ado to justify rejection of the diagnostic hypothesis (or hypotheses) for which "K" is inferable. A particular test result may be applicable in the effective elimination of multiple diagnostic possibilities. The general technique of elimination, as incorrect, of particular diagnostic hypotheses by falsification of their predictive consequences is of central importance in clinical diagnostic method. Notice that such falsification may affect not only diagnostic hypotheses but also "E", many conditions and assumptions, and law-statements in "K", serving an important role in enlarging and refining medical science.[21]

This technique is not always applicable, however, in such a relatively straightforward form, for many contexts do not permit the formulation of diagnostically useful strict (deductive) predictions.

"Probabilistic" Predictions

Consider now a similar framework of knowledge "K" and diagnostic hypotheses "h_a" and "h_b," a context in which the simple form of the eliminative technique just described is not applicable. This may come about in situations where no strict predictions are thus inferable, or where those that are inferable are equally so from "h_a" and "h_b", or where a potentially discriminatory strict prediction is not practically testable (in a given diagnostic context). In such situations, the clinician will ordinarily have recourse to the use of probabilistic predictions.

Such predictions may be made in various ways. They may be inferred from ordinary statistical laws or generalizations, in direct conformity with the inductive-statistical logical schema, or they may result from the use of universal law-statements in contexts where relevant antecedent conditions are not known definitely to be fulfilled, e.g., in the fringe of a range or where some needed information is uncertain or frankly unavailable. Recognized uncertainties surrounding causally relevant assumptions are carried through in the deductive uses of these laws in such contexts, the latter rendering their predictive conclusions only more or less probable. It has been argued that the predictive (and explanatory) uses of tendency laws can be usefully subjected to a similar analysis, where the strength attributed to a stated association of phenomena is seen to reflect the variable uncertainties in the satisfaction of other partially specifiable ante-cedent conditions. As has also been argued, the construal of either tendency laws or universal laws in contextually ill-fitting situations of use in merely statistical terms would seem distinctly misleading in respect to their underlying causal assumptions and certain important features in their use (e.g., the function of tendency-laws). Bearing earlier discussion in mind, the logic of clinical probabilistic predic-tions and their diagnostic uses will be further examined.

Consider first the use of a universal law statement in a context where there is explicit uncertainty in its applicability. In earlier ter-minology, the general deductive-nomological argument form may be expressed as follows:

(1) $\quad (C_1, C_2, \ldots C_k) . (L_1, L_2, \ldots L_r) \rightarrow E$

This may be re-written:

(2) $\quad (C_1, C_2, \ldots C_k) . L' \rightarrow E$

where the condensed "L'" represents a "minimal covering law" (termed by Hempel, and implied by but generally not equivalent to the conjunction from which it is derived), necessary for the validity of (2).[22] Joint truth in the statements ("C_i") of antecedent and boundary conditions, each (or most)[23] predicating some empiric property (e.g., "P_i"), is held on "L'" a sufficient condition for the truth of "E". The individual truth of each antecedent statement is commonly held also to be necessary for the truth of "E" in situations where "L'" is invoked, recognizing that "E" may be true on other grounds. Following earlier discussion, it is assumed that there are criteria, formulated in terms of kinds of evidential statements ("e_i") generally accepted as sufficient for the attribution of the various properties "P_i", permitting specifica-tion of a safe scope for "L'". Suppose now a situation of uncertainty in respect to the attribution of such a property, "P_j" (defined, say, as a range "R" of a variable), given the evidential statements "e_j" (e.g., describing a value of the variable near the edge of "R"), where other relevant conditions are held to be satisfied. (2) may now be amended in obvious ways to:

(3) $C_j \rightarrow (C'.L') \rightarrow E$

Probabilistically, what is of immediate interest here is:

(4) $p(E/C'.e_j')$

Inasmuch as $p(E/C'.C_j)$ would (on our suppositions) ordinarily receive the value "one," the value "r" assigned to (4) will accordingly be set equal to:

(5) $p(C_j/e_j')$

where the not exactly specifiable property "P_j" (predicated by "C_j") is understood to have some range of potential occasions for correct predication, beyond that implicit in its accepted criteria for attribution safe for "L'". Sufficient conditions for "P_j" are here more determinate in respect to the scope of "L'" than those that are necessary. The evidential statement "e_j'" may itself be understood to attribute a property, "P_j," although on our account this will not ordinarily correspond to an important clinical kind, within the concepts of accepted theory.

Following this terminology, (5) may be equated with:

(6) $p(P_j/P_j')$

where "P_j'" is construed as an uncertain instance of "K_j". A medical example of this relationship would be a white-blood-cell count of

3,900/mm^3 ("P$_j$'") as a possible instance of a normal white-blood-cell count ("P$_j$").

There are two main lines along which a clinician might in practice assign a value "r" to (4). On one hand, where there is minimal relevant theory and a good deal of related experience, her/his own or that reported by others, "r" might simply be identified with the observed relative frequency of truth among "E-type" statements derived in similar past situations.[24] Translated into a relation between properties (instead of between kinds of statements by which they are ascribed), (4) is on this hand conceived as an independent statistical hypothesis. This translation also permits subsumption of the use of such a hypothesis in an individual predictive (or explanation) instance within the inductive-statistical logical schema previously discussed.

She/he may, on the other hand, infer the value "r" of (4) from that assigned to (6). Situations in which "P$_j$" is largely statistically defined provide obvious examples, for example normal white blood cell count. Empiric reservations discussed concerning such statistical definitions should be kept in mind. However, "$p(P_j/P_j') = r$" may often instead be inferred from other accepted facts and theory, including higher-level statistical laws and generalizations. For instance, following an earlier example, let "P$_j$" be the property of having negligible (less than a certain threshold concentration, say) intrinsic factor in a patient with gastrectomy at time t_i, and "P$_j$'," having had a last previous dose of exogenous intrinsic factor at time t_i-0. Given available knowledge of average intestinal transit times etc., a clinician might (and could) infer the value of "$p(P_j/P_j')$". Numerous similar examples could be found in contexts (as in endocrinology, clinical pharmacology, nuclear medicine, etc.) involving consideration of the biological half-lives of endogenous or exogenous materials. On this method (6) and a fortiori (4) with assigned values must be regarded as theoretically derivative statistical hypotheses, in relation to which the observed relative frequency of successful "E-type" statements in similar past situations is construed merely as partial relevant evidence. It may be noted that use of "$p(P_j/P_j') = r$" in a particular predictive (or explanatory) instance can again be subsumed within the inductive-statistical schema. Several other comments concerning this account may now be made.

It is, first, no doubt true that values assigned to "r" will not be quantitatively exact. This has been not only recognized but also emphasized in previous discussion. However, such a value must be assigned at least within a roughly specified range or the predictions concerned would have little diagnostic (or other) use.

Second, the techniques suggested for the assignment of such values are to provide a substantially correct portrayal of accepted clinical methods. Clinicians would in general place little stock in probability estimates concerning individual events not involving at some point knowledge and use of statistical generalizations, informal and roughly quantitative as these may be, accepted as grounded either directly or indirectly (via the inferential use of other generalizations similarly grounded) in objective or subjective relative frequencies. This permits analysis of such estimates, whether and however they are associated with the use of universal or other law statements, by means of the inductive-statistical logical schema. It also permits corresponding adherence in their understanding to the notion of probability implicit in that model, an interpretation that seems best to conform to clinical concepts and practices. Clinical probability assignments commonly have important consequences—one or two such assignments can be determinative in diagnostic, therapeutic, and prognostic decision-making.

Third, where there are recognized uncertainties in the satisfaction of several antecedent conditions in the application of a universal law-statement, their effects on clinical probability estimates are generally treated (rightly or wrongly) as approximately multiplicative.

The justifying assumption of statistical independence would seem reasonable where there is no known, or theoretically surmised, causal relevance between the conditions concerned. Where there is knowledge of such causal relevance, clinicians may in such cases attempt to make rough adjustments in estimated probabilities. Importantly, in a situation where such uncertainties or the complexities of their joint effects become so rationally opaque that no reliable probability estimate (within a general range) can be derived, the prediction concerned would typically be abandoned as having no diagnostic (or other) usefulness. Clinicians tend to prudence in decision making.

Fourth, while it would appear on the present view that the probabilistic use of universal law-statements in contexts of their uncertain applicability can be analyzed with the aid of a statistical model, the uses of such laws in these (individual) cases in merely statistical terms would be misleading not only in respect to their causal assumptions but also in the role of any available causal knowledge. For the non-occurrence in such a case of a predicted event, whatever its assigned probability, it would be attributed not to mere chance (ultimate or inscrutable), but rather to the already suspected non-satisfaction of one or more specifiable antecedent causal conditions. The methodological import of this in respect to the utilization of such experience in the refinement of the law's scope (i.e., in the growth of knowledge) seems clear.

Finally, the relevance of the preceding discussion to the probabilistic predictions from tendency laws is apparent. Expression (3) might indeed be taken as the standard argument form for use of a tendency law, as these were earlier characterized. What is in question in such uses is again the (uncertain) satisfaction of some antecedent causal condition. Certain additional similarities and differences between use of such laws and that of (genuine) universal laws may be noted.

An obvious point of dissimilarity is that some antecedent condition(s) in a tendency law is not completely adequate for the law's uniform success. Given well-known difficulties in biological measurement, and assessment of such clinically important properties as "functional immune system," this problematic element of unspecifiability may reflect only insufficient determinateness in available criteria for attribution of certain conditions recognized to be among relevant antecedents.[25] (Bear in mind that these may be complex properties, perhaps exhibiting complex causal interrelationships). On the other hand, certain such antecedent factors may not yet have been defined or their importance recognized. In either case,[26] while there is explicit uncertainty only occasionally in the use of an accepted universal law, whose safe scope is at least sometimes held to be satisfied, such uncertainty will be indigenous in the use of a tendency law for which a safe scope, so long as it remains unconverted, is ex *hypothesi* not yet fully determinate. Conceived as an incompletely formulated causal law, there will be within a given state of knowledge a roughly appreciated probability of a tendency law's failure, as a quasi-universal, even when used in situations seen as relatively optimal for its applicability. This probability must be appropriately reckoned with in the law's variously less optimal situations of use, whose analysis may then be further understood in conformity with the above account. Difficulties that may sometimes surround attribution of properties with greater than usual vagueness in their specification must be recognized. There may again be instances of joint uncertainties concerning the satisfaction of several antecedent conditions of known causal relevance. Such complexities as may occur cannot justifiably be swept aside, but neither should the importance of such complexities be exaggerated. In most contexts of use of such laws in medicine there would be little doubt concerning the satisfaction of most such antecedents, with fair agreement generally obtainable in the satisfaction of others. Importantly, again, when such complexities are considered to render impossible the assignment of a reliable probability to a prediction based on the use of some such law, clinicians would as a rule regard the prediction as having little or no diagnostic or other usefulness.[27]

A further important similarity between the use of a tendency law and that of uncertainly applied universal laws, already remarked on, rests in the manner of treatment of their failures. An apparent failure of a tendency law would be regularly analyzed first in relation to the possible non-satisfaction of antecedent conditions of known causal relevance, and attributed only as a last resort to the (yet) unreduced element of chance in its usage.[28] The major methodological importance of this in clinical medicine, in the uncovering of abnormalities and the elucidation of means for their testing, and in the ongoing refinement of pertinent causal knowledge.[28]

There are, certainly, instances of probabilistic prediction in medicine that conform in a relatively straightforward manner with use of the inductive-statistical logical schema. Those which do so need no further comment here.[29] However, a point may be brought out concerning the possible use of this argument form in more complex situations where there is available considerable relevant causal knowledge—i.e., where a tendency law might become appropriate.

It may be thought that the potential complexities in usage of a tendency law, particularly respecting the need and use of complex evidence, might be avoided by merely falling back onto the use of an ordinary (simpler) inductive-statistical form of argument. This would seem, however, a mistaken supposition. Whatever evidence there is relating to the possible satisfaction of antecedents of known causal relevance in a tendency law argument should clearly fall within the compass of the total available relevant evidence whose use is methodologically required in an acceptable corresponding inductive-statistical argument.[30] The latter will therefore be at least no less complex in its evidential base, at a given time, than the former. This evidential base is in practice moreover not ordinarily fixed once and for all, and it seems clear that failure of a probabilistic argument—whatever its form—to take account of evidence relevant to its conclusion must lessen its practical adequacy. A tendency law construal helps to elucidate, in this regard, the notion previously set forth that an acceptable probabilistic prediction (or explanation) in clinical medicine should be based on evidence appropriately complete in respect to information of recognized potential relevance to its reasoning. Such evidence is that which in an individual context is practically obtainable (without undue risk, etc.) and seen to be important in relation to the possible satisfaction of known causal antecedents. Satisfaction of a particular antecedent—e.g., a normal immune function—is often simply assumed. However, when there is evidence that it might not be satisfied, or when the prediction (or explanation) concerned is of especial importance, additional relevant evidence would ordinarily be demanded, and selectively acquired, as part of an acceptable probabilistic argument.[31]

A tendency law analysis of such arguments, with its suggested manner of acquisition and use of evidence in appraisal of the possible satisfaction of generally identifiable causal antecedent conditions, provides a thorough and more accurate account of most probabilistic inference in clinical medicine, as currently practiced, than would a merely (black box) statistical model, relating to individual cases with their multitudinous particular attributes. Medical—and particularly clinical—investigation has naturally focused on the causal relationships between such clinically important biological properties (common end points in clinical reasoning) as diseases and their properties. Given a good deal of success in this, i.e., growing knowledge of causal linkages, an attempted general representation of probabilistic inference containing reference to such properties in purely statistical terms would seem frankly implausible, becoming increasingly so as such inferences gain in causal refinement. Along with its important methodological implications, a tendency law construal serves better to explicate the structure of most such inferences, providing a useful conceptual bridge between those more basic argument forms that may be regarded as either simply statistical or mundanely deductive. It would seem reasonable to see this as corresponding to a normal route of evolution (in use) of multiplying general causal laws in medical science.

Clearly, adjustments in the relative probability assignments of alternative diagnostic hypotheses with accumulating evidence must involve at least tacit use of some set of principles (transformation rules) regulating such inferential transactions. Those that are implicit in generally accepted clinical method are very much like those commonly invoked elsewhere in science, and in respect to most practical affairs of everyday life. Methods used may vary somewhat between clinicians and between contexts. Bearing in mind too that clinicians do not generally deal with numerically exact probabilities, and that our purpose is an elucidation of clinical method as it is used—and not as it should or could be if knowledge were more perfect—a rather loose characterization of these principles must suffice. In our previous terminology, and with the assumption that a diagnostic hypothesis "h_d" while remaining under consideration will be accorded a finite probability of truth, the principles of interest may be formulated as follows.

(i)   The observed success or failure of a given probabilistic prediction based on "h_d" (with "K") will be regarded respectively as confirmatory or disconfirmatory of that hypothesis (acceptance of the relevant knowledge-state "K" into which new evidence is incorporated having been supposed).

(ii)   The extent to which "h_d" will be regarded as thus confirmed (or disconfirmed) by the success (or failure) of a given prediction will vary in roughly direct proportion with the strength (probability) attributed to the prediction on the supposition of "h_d" (with "K").

(iii) The confirmatory effects of several successful predictions from "h_d" will be more or less strongly reinforcing in their joint effect.

(iv) The relation expressed in (iii) will analogously hold for the joint disconfirmatory effect of several failed predictions.

The confirmation of "h_d" (a singular proposition) is understood here in correspondence with its probability assigned in relation to the class of accepted statements "K". Principles (i)-(iv), which seem intuitive and generally accepted at least in clinical decision-making, will be recognized as broadly consonant with a Bayesian strategy of probabilistic inference. They will be elaborated, with other pertinent matters, in relation to a more explicitly and formally Bayesian analysis in a later section. However, an informal representation of these relationships better captures the quantitatively inexact (and mathematically unrefined) manner of their use in clinical diagnosis.

Given then that (with "K" assumed) the failure of a probabilistic prediction from a certain diagnostic hypothesis will not entail the falsity of the hypothesis, the latter will yet be regarded as disconfirmed by such a failure to an extent varying in rough proportion with the probability (or strength) ascribed to the prediction on the supposition of the hypothesis concerned.[32] In practice, the failure of a single prediction held very probable in relation to a given diagnostic hypothesis (e.g., as might follow use of the tuberculin skin test in a context considered optimal for the satisfaction of other causal conditions of known relevance) is often taken to effectively rule out the corresponding disease. Alternatively, the joint failures of several different predictions will commonly have the same result for a diagnostic hypothesis in relation to which they are individually held fairly probable, etc. In any case, evidence selectively disconfirmatory for a particular diagnostic hypothesis will be seen to increase the relative probability of an alternative diagnostic hypothesis still under consideration.

On the suppositions of our simplified case, concerning the initially reasonably probable differential diagnostic hypotheses, "h_a" (here assumed correct) and "h_b" (assumed incorrect), it may be expected that most of the subsequently tested strong predictions from "h_a" will succeed and that many of the predictions from "h_b," weak and strong, will fail. In particular, those predictions from "h_b" should fail that are in that context not also predictions from "h_a". The methodological importance of the clinician's selective testing of those predictions that in the given situation most sharply distinguish between the alternative diagnostic hypotheses under consideration is clear. Complex as clinical diagnosis may be in respect to the number of diagnostic hypotheses considered, and the knowledge and inference brought to bear in their evaluation, the clinician's selection between any two such alternatives typically turns on the acquisition and use of only a few key items of evidence seen most decisively to upset the balance of their relative probabilities.

The process of selection between diagnostic hypotheses by means of their differential testing may involve more or less patient discomfort, risk, cost, and time. Evidence from such things as clinical course and response to a therapeutic trial may be needed. At best, given available knowledge and technology, it is not always successful; the imperfections in an imperfect science must be recognized.

These matters will be pursued further in subsequent sections, beginning with some typical complicating factors in the more general case.

The General Case

The usual case of diagnosis selection variously involves a number of complexities not so far examined. It has been pointed out that the clinician must evaluate evidence not only against diagnostic hypotheses newly considered, but must relate both such evidence and diagnostic hypotheses to the patient's previously diagnosed diseases and/ or conditions. Certain additional complexities that commonly beset the more general diagnostic situation will now be brought out.

Simple and compound hypotheses

As was earlier remarked a particular diagnostic hypothesis "h_d" may be composite (or compound). This qualification is needed on our analysis in relation to the common clinical situation in which a patient presents with more than one previously undiagnosed disease.[33]

Co-existing diseases (or conditions) may exhibit all manner of causal inter-relations. They may be seen as separately identifiable aspects of a more general condition or disease, e.g., cerebrovascular disease and coronary artery disease in relation to generalized arteriosclerosis, or as joint effects of another (perhaps complex) disease (e.g., osteomalacia, renal lithiasis, and duodenal ulcer in relation to hyper-parathyroidism; relapsing pancreatitis and hepatic cirrhosis in relation to alcoholism; peripheral neuropathy and glomerulosclerosis in relation to diabetes mellitus; etc.), or one of two suspected diseases may be seen simply as a probable effect of the other (e.g., any of the above effect conditions in relation to the causal one; pulmonary infarction in relation to thrombophlebitis; etc.). Or, co-existing diseases may be deemed causally non-related (e.g., duodenal ulcer and otitis media).

Certain diseases may thus in individual contexts be regarded as either primary or secondary (et cetera) states, depending on their accepted causal relations with other conditions also diagnosed. Assessment of such potentially complex relationships between diseases and their effects in particular cases may involve a process of causal inference and testing of considerable intricacy.

Although a secondary disease (or condition) will then properly be regarded as evidential in relation to certain other (causally anteced-ent) diagnostic possibilities, it will itself figure causally in the genera-tion of a further class of effects (e.g., as in pneumococcal pneumonia secondary to an obstructive bronchogenic carcinoma),[34] to which diagnostic and therapeutic attention must appropriately relate. Such conditions are therefore typically regarded as more or less discretely identifiable components of a more complex total disease state, the latter being correspondingly characterized by means of a compound proposition built up from the clinician's stock of accepted diagnostic predicates (e.g., "arteriosclerotic heart disease with myocardial infarc-tion and congestive heart failure," etc.).

The nature and uses of these fairly distinctive but not rigidly demarcated predicates has been discussed.[35] Suppose the clinician's class of such accepted predicates to be represented by "D_1, D_2, ... D_n". Then, in the framework of this analysis, a particular diagnostic hypothesis "h_d" may employ any sub-set (ordinarily a small number) or logically compatible members of this class.[36] It may, that is, be simple or compound in its utilization of such predicates. A com-pound "h_d", which may be understood as a combination diagnosis, is potentially entertained, tested, and selected in a manner generally parallel with that of a simple case. Certain further observations on such diagnoses and their use may now be made.

It should be seen that diagnostic conditions denoted by such predicates having recognized causal interrelationships will not in general be statistically independent. With an eye to roughly known relative frequencies as the most commonly accepted determinants of such initial probabilities, the conjunction of two fairly improbable conditions—myocardial infarction and congestive heart failure, say, where the latter may be an effect of the former—need not be, by a correspondingly rough use of the multiplication axiom, very improbable. Moreover, the extent of statistical independence between such conditions will vary with the possible additional presence of other causally associated diseases, e.g., coronary artery disease, of which both of the above may be effects. Hence, a particular diagnostic hypothesis need not be assigned an unusually low initial probability merely because it is compound, and the clinician's assignment of such a rough probability would ordinarily take at least implicit account of recognized causal relationships between the several conditions predicated.

Second, given the often interwoven causal relationships between co-present diseases and their manifestations, as these are commonly characterized, it should not be supposed that a body of evidence, "E*," (including such manifestations) will regularly be divisible into parts to which components in a compound diagnosis may be separately related. Such compartmentalization of diagnostic conditions and their manifestations may at times be practicable (e.g., as with otitis media and duodenal ulcer), but it will often not be, for such conditions jointly present commonly interact as causal antecedents in their manifestations—as a patient with pneumonia and dehydration may fail to exhibit the usual auscultatory rales, etc. Such interactions prevent a general analysis of the logic of use of compound diagnostic propositions in terms of separately independent parts, invoking only simple one-to-one relations between conditions predicated and differentiable classes of clinically characterized manifestations. This consideration supports the accuracy as well as the convenience of the present treatment of such propositions as particular diagnostic hypotheses.[37]

Third, insofar as a diagnostic predicate is of any use, its addition to a given diagnostic hypothesis ("h_j") will ordinarily augment the logical explanatory and predictive strength of the latter, potentially converting an inadequate "h_j" into an adequate "h_k" in relation to available evidence "E*". However, this added logical strength may clearly be a liability as well as an asset, for it may lead to strongly disconfirmatory false predictions on subsequent testing. Clinicians do not then attempt to salvage inadequate diagnoses by mere ad hoc additions of predicates. Compound diagnoses are tested as rigorously as simple ones; they may indeed be tested more rigorously, inasmuch as each condition ascribed carries some of its own prognostic implications and therapeutic demands. Clinicians therefore adhere to a principle of economy in their use of such predicates, selecting the simplest (if sometimes compound) diagnostic hypothesis that meets other conditions for acceptance.[38]

Fourth, the abandonment of a particular compound diagnostic hypothesis clearly does not require the rejection of each, or if the hypothesis is logically too weak rather than too strong, of any of its component diagnostic predicates. A patient with a suspected diagnosis of coronary artery disease (CAD) and congestive heart failure (CHF) may eventually be diagnosed instead as myocarditis (or aortic valvular disease, etc.) and CHF. Alternatively, the eventual diagnosis might be CAD and chronic obstructive pulmonary disease (COPD). The final diagnosis might also be the conjunction of CAD, CHF, and COPD. All of these clinically commonplace diagnostic possibilities are also commonly differential alternatives in individual cases. Whether introduced for consideration <u>de novo</u> or as amendments of other possibilities, though, particular diagnostic hypotheses are subject to a similar process of testing of their net logical consequences in their candidature for selection.

Finally, it is certainly true that not all clinical diagnoses are thus compound. Simple diagnoses (e.g., streptococcal pharyngitis) are, in certain classes of patients, the rule. There are other classes of patients, e.g., the aged or the seriously ill, where troubles tend to mount quickly, and in the causal ways suggested to multiply. In such patients, compound diagnostic hypotheses are more often called for, in relation to evidence in question, than not. A general account of the clinical diagnostic process must therefore include attention to the role and manner of use of these more complex propositions.

Multiple Hypotheses

It was assumed in the simplified case discussion above that the clinician's list of differential diagnoses contained just two diagnostic hypotheses. In practice, such a list would often include several such members. However, the process of selection between any pair of diagnostic possibilities should be sequentially applicable to any longer list, so that used order of this assumption to cover that the general case would appear to raise no special logical difficulties.

More problematic, however, is relaxation of the assumption, tentatively made above, that one of the members of the accepted list of differential diagnoses should be correct. In the usual case, of course, the clinician is not entitled to this assumption. It may be that she/he has simply failed to consider a known disease (condition or disorder) that is in fact present. This is especially apt to occur when the disease is rare or present in a highly atypical form. It may also depend on a failure on whatever basis to uncover important relevant evidence—the importance of a thorough preliminary examination and the use of screening tests is apparent. The many different diseases now characterized in relation to each organ, or organ system, and the much greater number of their possible combinations is worth remembering. Clinicians do not assume, moreover, that all naturally occurring diseases have indeed been thus characterized, i.e., that available diagnostic predicates must in all possible cases suffice in the formulation of adequate (correct) diagnoses, or new such predicates would not be introduced as they are from time to time.

Clinicians may then sometimes arrive at an errant diagnosis through failure to consider, for whatever reason, the correct one. Importantly, they sometimes arrive at no (genuine) diagnosis, particularly in situations where all diagnostic possibilities considered have failed to stand up to the clinician's satisfaction, to appropriate testing.[39]

As a clinician may assign approximate probabilities (high, low, etc.) to individual diagnostic hypotheses, she/he may also assign a perhaps rougher probability to a particular disjunction of such hypotheses. Given a manageably small set of reasonably probable alternatives, as would ordinarily come into consideration in a diagnostic context, the probability assigned to their disjunction might be more or less high, being at least no less than that assigned to its most probable member. As a corollary of the above, the clinician may not assume in respect to a list of differential diagnoses that the individual probabilities of its member hypotheses should sum no more than one. Correspondingly, a particular diagnosis is not generally accepted merely by the ruling out of those several diagnoses considered initially its most probable rivals. Such acceptance normally requires further that a diagnosis must itself have met the challenges of testing—i.e., that it should not itself be ruled out. A diagnosis eventually selected as correct may have been first considered late in the diagnostic process, after the practical rejection of many earlier alternatives, or sometimes none is selected, more often early in the process.

Diseases are not always presented to the clinician for diagnosis in a natural (pristine) form, however typical or atypical this might be. The manifestations of a disease in a given case may have been more or less radically altered by a variety of intervening factors. In particular, they may have been altered by earlier medical treatment. For example, a patient with subacute bacterial endocarditis might exhibit normal blood (bacteriological) cultures if recently given antibiotic treatment for an upper respiratory infection. Certain diagnostic conditions, e.g., Cushing's syndrome, are themselves recognized to be in some instances the iatrogenic effects of medical treatment. Thus, the clinician must take into account the possible effects of medical therapy known to have been previously administered, by whomever and for whatever, in relating available evidence to the diagnostic hypotheses.

Methodological Comments

First, events described, or properties ascribed, are understood as events or properties of certain "kinds". For the clinician these kinds may be such things as positive or negative tuberculin skin test reactions, normal or enlarged heart size, etc., encompassing certain (inexactly specified) ranges, or agreed upon varieties of phenomena. Abnormal ranges are commonly subdivided into a few narrower ranges, corresponding to several recognized grades—constituent kinds—of the abnormality. For example, a tuberculin skin test reaction may be weakly or strongly positive, a heart size may be slightly, moderately or massively enlarged, the intensity of a heart murmur may range from grade 1/6 to grade 6/6 (in conventional terminology), etc. (cf. also such further standard characterizations of heart murmurs as systolic or diastolic, decrescendo or diamond-shaped, high-pitched or rumbling, and so on.) Abnormal ranges of continuous variables are commonly graded in a similar way, as clinicians would routinely describe an abnormal serum enzyme value as slightly, moderately or highly elevated. Other terms are used also, e.g., in a "1-plus" to "4-plus" scale of abnormality.

It may be noted again that although conditions for application of terms like those above are not exactly specifiable, good agreement would be found among clinicians concerning their acceptable use, and little practical doubt would surround most of their actual occasions of use. It might also be surmised that relevant kinds of phenomena would be differently characterized. In situations where there is doubt—e.g., when evidence is seen as borderline and the matter is consequential, e.g., "is this a positive-tuberculin skin test reaction," or "is that a significant 1-plus systolic murmur,"—clinicians typically treat the evidence as inadequate and repeat the test, confer with other observers, etc., until the question of which kind term(s) should apply is considered reliably decidable.[40]

The qualifying "most" is needed because the confirmatory or disconfirmatory effect of a certain finding will depend on temporal considerations, as elevated cardiac serum markers would confirm the diagnosis of acute myocardial infarction at a few hours after the event but disconfirm it at a few days later, if unknown temporal events.[41] Similarly, the presence of other causally relevant conditions, as absence of auscultatory rales at an appropriate time would be strongly disconfirmatory of pneumococcal pneumonia, but much less so in a severely dehydrated patient.

In sum, what confirms a particular diagnostic hypothesis in an individual patient context is the accepted instantiation, on the evidence, of the kinds of phenomena that could be inferred (expected) on the supposition of that hypothesis in that context, with consideration of temporal relations, other conditions present, previously administered treatment, etc., while the evident failures of such instantiations are conversely disconfirmatory of it. Most kinds of evidence are not held to stand, as in fact many do not, usual attempts at the formulation of diagnostic algorithms notwithstanding, in individually constant relations with particular diseases.[42]

The topics discussed in this section are aimed at major sorts of complexity encountered in the general diagnostic process. Given its monumental intricacy, their analysis is seen to fit within an account of diagnosis on the hypotheses-inferential model, a framework that is more able than others to illuminate the nature and manner of treatment of such complexities in the process of medical diagnosis.

REFERENCES AND FOOTNOTES: CHAPTER 7

1. Cabot, R.C., Differential Diagnosis, Op cit., p. 19.
2. Stanley D., and Campos D., Op cit., pp 300-308.
3. Eddy D., NEJM Vol 306 No 21 May 27, 1982, "The art of diagnosis." pp 1263-1268
4. Barrows H. S., Clinical and Investigative Medicine Vol 5:1 1982 "The clinical reasoning of randomly selected physicians in general medical practice." pp 49-55
5. Croskerry P., Canadian Journal Anesthesiology 2005: 52:6 "The theory and practice of clinical decision-making" pp R1-R8 In a study of evident research, this author reports "Over 60% of lead authors for the 51 articles published in medical decision-making in 2004 were not physicians." p R3. This may have reflected the surge in articles dealing with statistics and psychology.
6. Sisson J. C., Academic Medicine Volume 66 Number 10 Oct. 1991, "The Characteristics of Early Diagnostic Hypotheses Generated by Physicians (Experts) and Students (Novices) at One Medical School." pp 607-612
7. Cabot, Op cit, p. 18.
8. McCaughan D., (2008) Transactions of the Charles S. Peirce Society, v. 44, no. 3 (summer)"From Ugly Duckling to Swan. C. S. Peirce, Abduction and the Pursuit of Scientific Theories." pp 446-468
9. Cf. the clinical saw: "when you hear hoofbeats (in N. America, say), don't think first of a giraffe!"
10. Cabot, Op cit, p19
11. In "potential explanation" it should be understood that some allowance will be made for imperfect knowledge ("could disease 'A' under these conditions result in manifestation 'x'?") as will come out in later discussion. It should also be noted that on our suppositions the singular statements comprising "E*" will be included in "K" and therefore

trivially inferable from "$_{Hd.K}$". But this will not count as their explana-tion in respect either to the covering-law model or to common usage where (as said before) a given manifestation of disease is not permitted to figure in its own explanation. A certain manifestation might, however, be referred to in an explanation of some other manifestation, i.e., some statements in "E^*" might be explanatorily relevant to other such statements.

12. This might be seen as a common working assumption in the compila-tion and use of such lists. Although it would usually be regarded as only tentative, the assumption is connected with the requirement that the initial formulation of a list of differential diagnoses should be reasonably comprehensive, including diagnostic possibilities which based on preliminary information might be deemed quite improbable. Despite this, such a hypothesis may be included because of high risk (e.g., EBOLA). The advantages of an early inclusion among those actively considered are apparent.

13. Contextual considerations, e.g., the relative threats to the patient, or others, as in possible contagion of the given disease possibilities, the potential benefits and risks of their respective treatments, the risks and costs of further available test procedures pertinent to their discrimina-tion, etc. While clinicians would rarely venture the assignment of numerical probability values to diagnostic hypotheses, even after extensive testing, they commonly come to agree, after a similar process of testing, on the general ranges of such values and their relations (e.g., "much more probable"), as used in diagnosis selection.

14. The need for such information was discussed in relation to the accept-ability of probabilistic explanations in clinical medicine. Given the importance of a correct diagnosis, and the view of various diagnostic hypotheses as providing in conjunction with the clinician's knowledge alternative explanatory accounts of the evidence of disease, the require-ment for a high degree of evidential completeness, in the indicated respect, in the selection of an acceptable (presumably "correct")

account is clearly appropriate. Most such explanatory accounts will indeed by "probabilistic," conforming to the usual relation between a disease and any particular set of its case manifestations <u>in toto</u>, "E*". It may also be noted that the acquisition of such information must as a rule be accompanied by the clinician's increased preference for the actually correct diagnosis (or the diagnostic process would not generally work). This general condition then compliments the first.

15. Practical doubts concerning this are usually resolved in clinical diagnosis, as elsewhere in science, by repeat testing.

16. Understanding this here and elsewhere to mean: "hi in conjunction with 'K'."

17. This is changing with new knowledge of causal linkages between test findings – such as genetic abnormalities -- and diseases.

18. Croskerry P., Canadian Journal Anesthesiology 2005: 52:6"The theory and practice of clinical decision-making" Pages R1-R8

19. Berner E., The American Journal of Medicine 2008 volume 121 (5A) "Overconfidence as a cause of diagnostic error in medicine." pages S2-S23

20. Croskerry P., The American Journal of Medicine" (2008) volume 121 (5A) "Over-confidence in Clinical Decision-Making" pages S24-S29

21. These dynamics and their fruits will be further discussed later.

22. Hempel, <u>Aspects of Scientific Explanation</u>, pp. 346-47.
The notion of a "minimal covering law" relates to the familiar use of "condensed" deductive argument forms as previously discussed, in which a number of laws (and some initial and boundary conditions) are tacitly assumed in the formulation of clinically convenient law-statements relating important and commonly encountered properties of the organism (e.g., "Every person who has a total gastrectomy soon develops defective vitamin B_{12} absorption"). "L" in the above discussion should be understood as some such law-statement. Additionally, the term "minimal" above should not be over-emphasized or too strong. Given wider scope for probabilistic

inference, from another perspective this covering law model has more utility in medical science, whether or not being "stronger."

23. Depending on whether "E" is taken to ascribe a property or describe an event. The referents of most statements of antecedent conditions in the use of such a law can more easily be understood as "properties" (e.g., "disease states") than as "events." Many biological law statements may themselves be similarly construed as co-relating properties of organisms (e.g., "all persons with insulin deficiency have abnormal carbohydrate metabolism.") But an argument analogous to the above could be given in terms of (kinds of) "events." Cf. D. H. Mellor, "The Matter of Chance" Cambridge, UK, Cambridge Univ. Press (1971), p. 170.

24. Using, as clinicians regularly do, a so-called "straight-rule" of inductive inference. For discussion of such rules see M. Hesse. Op cit., p. 91 and passim.

25. Reference among such criteria to the event whose prediction is in question (as a positive tuberculin skin test would be evidence of a functional immune system) may obviously complicate the predictive use of a tendency law -- or of any other law. But such reference is usually only partial -- there are other independent criteria; in our example, a positive mumps skin test, etc., and the absence of corresponding evidence would rarely present a major difficulty in such prediction.

26. These alternative possibilities are clearly not independently resolvable, and a decision between them might sometimes be difficult ("could there be a 'hidden variable'?"). But the difficulty is practically more apparent than real, for the matter would ordinarily be at least tentatively decided on the basis of available related knowledge, e.g., in the association between hyperlipidemia, cigarette smoking, hypertension, etc., on the one hand, and coronary artery disease on the other could be seen as reflecting the influence of still unrecognized causal factors (another example of this type would be the relation between environmental conditions and malignancy, etc.). Clearly, either kind

of problem should be to at least some extent amenable to improved knowledge and techniques.

27. An exception to this rule might be the prediction of an event accepted as highly specific, or even "pathognomonic," for a particular disease. Its occurrence would accordingly be taken in most contexts as diagnostically decisive no matter how strongly, weakly, or uncertainly it might have been predicted (or predictable -- it may have been quite unforeseen) simply because it could not be explained or predicted on the basis of any other disease hypothesis. We have seen, however, that such events are not common within kinds of evidence available in clinical diagnosis. Neither, as a matter of interest to our account, is their observation commonly fortuitous.

28. Invoking again the tendency law construal as a "quasi-universal," whereas statistical laws do not in individual instances "fail."

29. It is of interest to note, however, that clinical probabilistic arguments are commonly formulated in subjunctive or counter-factual form: e.g., "If Mr. Jones has (had) streptococcal pharyngitis, it would very probably respond (have responded) to penicillin," etc. This is consistent with the present account of the logic and diagnostic uses of such arguments.

30. The requirement for use of such evidence is satisfyingly implicit in tendency law usage, as in that of ordinary universal laws, and need not be attached as an independent methodological rider.

31. It should not be imagined that the assigned probabilities of predictions in individual cases, involving such arguments, hover in the vicinity of a statistical mean. Depending on the assessed satisfaction of recognized causal antecedents, a given kind of prediction (describing, for example, a positive tuberculin skin test) may be assigned probability values (ranges) from practically zero to near unity.

32. Inasmuch as the hypothesis would be regarded as confirmed by success of the prediction, this corresponds to a lemma of elementary confirmation theory.

33. O'Connor, P., JAMA, August 10, 2005 Vol 294 No 06, "Adding Value to Evidence-Based Clinical Guidelines." pp 741-743

34. The disease pneumococcal pneumonia is commonly involved in the relation under consideration. While often diagnosed in a "primary" form, it is also recognized as a common consequence of various other ("predisposing") diseases.

35. Although certainly restricted within the larger class of medical descriptive terms such predicates are not bound in common clinical usage to a narrow or fixed sense of "disease." "Myocardial infarction" and "congestive heart failure" are regularly accepted clinical diagnoses (as is "laceration"). Hence the occasional use above of the more neutral "condition" respecting the referents of such predicates.

36. The conjunction of definitionally contradictory predicates would of course be barred (e.g., "hyperthyroidism" and "hypothyroidism"), and other conjunctions might be nearly so for reasons of relative theoretic incompatibility (e.g., "Addison's disease" and "essential hypertension").

37. Where disease possibilities jointly entertained as parts of a combination diagnosis are believed to be causally independent, in respect to each other and each other's effects, they may be separately diagnosed (in relation to segmental evidence) in a sequential fashion. This may also happen when a particular disease is independently diagnosed based on specific (or "pathognomonic") evidence. But this is as above not always feasible, and does not in any case greatly complicate our account, which will then concern the structure of diagnosis selection in relation to the evidence segment "E*", etc.

38. The clinician's intuitively desirable parsimony in this regard can be defended on logical grounds, in respect to the exclusion of explanatorily irrelevant or redundant diagnostic predicates. Suppose, for example, that alternative diagnostic hypotheses "h_j" and "h_k" differ only by inclusion in the latter of "D_k" (assuming, in knowledge-state "K", that "h_j" and "h_k" are and remain logically inequivalent, i.e., that "D_k" is not entailed in "K" by use of other predicates in "h_j"), and that

"Dk" confers no useful added explanatory strength on "hk" above that of "hj", in relation to evidence available through the time of diagnosis selection. Inasmuch as the "initial probability" assigned to "Dk" is less than unity, the initial probability assigned to "hk" should (on our assumptions) be at least somewhat lower than that of "hj". Supposing further only that whatever "transformation rule" used by the clinician in the assignment of "posterior" probabilities is used without bias, the ratio of their assigned probabilities should continue to favor "hj" at every step in their testing, resulting in the selection (if either) of the simpler hypothesis "hj".

39. Resort is commonly made in such situations to quasi-diagnostic descriptive phrases detailing certain signs, symptoms, etc. (e.g., "transient mid-abdominal pain," or "intermittent dizziness," etc., perhaps with the addendum: "etiology undetermined"). The differences between such phrases and diagnoses (e.g., "duodenal ulcer"), with their explanatory and predictive uses should be clear.

40. This is usually possible. If in a given case its applicability continues to be regarded uncertain, on all available evidence, inferential use of such a term would be correspondingly probabilistic, if its probability is considered sufficiently determinate to warrant any such inferential use.

41. Boersma, E., The Lancet Vol 361 March 8, 2003, "Acute myocardial infarction." pp 847-858

42. Groopman, J., Op cit., p. 5

CHAPTER 8

Ramifications

Introduction

It was suggested earlier that a general understanding of clinical diagnostic methods should have a useful bearing on a number of other issues relating to the physician's status and work. Many of these are controversial subjects of recurrent debate. While they are matters largely outside the scope of this essay, a few subjects might yet be of interest based on implications having to do with the present account. Some disclaimers of this account will also be discussed.

Ramifications

Testing: Positive and Negative Results

Confirmatory and disconfirmatory functions of evidence, as related to possible diagnoses, were seen as logically complimentary in the clinical diagnostic process. The importance of evidence seen as having a disconfirmatory role (whether corresponding to normal or abnormal findings), in the rejection of incorrect diagnostic possibilities, has long been recognized in medical practice. It is recognized implicitly in the common use of various screening tests (e.g., the tuberculin skin test, etc.). It is often recognized in medical literature dealing with practical problems in diagnosis, most plainly in relation to what are known as "diagnoses by exclusion." Clinicians have, in short, appreciated in practice that the usefulness of evidence does not depend just on its having direct confirmatory import for specific disease possibilities.[1-5]

While clinicians understand and use disconfirmatory (negative) evidence in diagnostic logic, confirmatory evidence may tend to capture the eye; the real thing (or not) may bring a bias to the most plausible, but not the only source of this evidence. The experienced and wary clinician would avoid such a decision until all relevant needed evidence is available. The needed kind of evidence stems from the clinician's knowledge and judgment as the testing proceeds (over several hours or days, etc.) in the patient's individual case.

A larger issue on this topic exists outside clinicians and other medical scientists, e.g., some businesses at the fringes of clinical medicine. Interested outside parties too often regard negative diagnostic tests to be unnecessary, neglecting the important role of disconfirmatory evidence. To some extent, this issue is widespread within our society.

Point: A quotation by B. Berghman and H. C. Schouten: "My hypothesis is that in medical schools and education no, or insufficient, attention is being given to the philosophy of science in general, and Popper's theory in particular."[6]

Medical Investigation: Human Experimentation

While ethical and legal issues surrounding the subject of human experimentation in medicine are but a small part in our topic, a brief comment on this matter should be in order. A more general but also brief discussion of medical ethics will follow.

The logical and practical intimacy in the association between "investigative" and "applied" activities within clinical medicine has been previously emphasized. Many of these activities involve elements of what cannot but be called human experimentation. These would most clearly include the use of innovative techniques in medical testing, or the introduction of new modes of treatment; virtually all forms of accepted treatment would at one time have fit into this category. However, inasmuch as individual cases are always in some respects novel, and clinicians view their knowledge as comprising only variously reliable and revisable scientific generalizations (and not as a compendium of dogma), there is a sense in which the clinical handling of every patient is, or might be considered, in some degree experimental.[7] Individual case observations and reports (as might concern, for example, unusual diseases, or sporadic and/or delayed side effects of accepted kinds of treatment), reflecting clinical experience at an ordinary level, have contributed significantly to the growth of medical knowledge; the importance in this of the clinician's scientific curiosity should not be overlooked.[8]

Clinical freedoms in the exercise of human experimentation are certainly far from absolute, being strictly subject to a variety of constraints, having to do with informed and voluntary patient consent, the minimizing of risk and its relation to expected gain, etc. The importance and propriety of some such constraints is not in question. What might be questioned, however, is the tenability of the view, sometimes expressed, that conventional and currently accepted constraints on clinical experimentation should be greatly expanded, codified in much finer detail, or indeed that such experimentation should be altogether proscribed.

The general effect of such a proscription, if written, would be as broadly undesirable as foreseeable; the stultification of medical science. Not only would there result a stagnation (spreading from the clinical level) of overt medical research, but clinicians would in general be driven into a defensive posture of dogmatic traditionalism, eschewing the use of anything new or unconventional in diagnostic or treatment methods. What object might reasonably be taken to warrant so high a price? Not the collective interest of society. Would many wish that such a ban, creating a milieu in which it would be difficult to imagine the survival of a scientific spirit, had been imposed at some earlier time in the development of modern medicine? But neither could it be—at least in any obvious way—the interests or rights of individual patients. Have patients with diseases whose medical management is largely ineffective, within a given framework of knowledge and technology, no interest in or right to new approaches that offer some possible gain, if not to themselves then perhaps to others? May individual patients have no legitimate interest here, as well as risk? To whom, if not clinicians, might hold primary responsibility for the conception, introduction, testing, and use of new diagnostic and therapeutic measures, with assessment of their relative risks and benefits for living human beings in various states of health and disease, reasonably be entrusted?

Perhaps an outright proscription of this kind is not, indeed, a serious possibility, but its probable consequences might be approached, and a similar if less extreme state of affairs reached by other routes. Conceivably, clinicians could just lose interest in advancing their science. More plausibly, their ability and willingness to advance might be lost through erosion of privileges vital for progress in science. This might come about if remedies for recognized abuse (within the terms of current law and common morality) of human experimentation in medicine were sought not so much in the rectification, insofar as possible, of such occurrences (by reasonable compensation for injuries, punishment of offenders, etc.) as in improved new measures for their prevention. Can then the potential for abuse of a privilege be effectively eliminated without abrogation of the privilege itself?

Suppose these preventive measures were to involve the operation of agencies empowered with the regulation of all such experimentation at a detailed practical level, in accordance with finely specific codes, etc. Wouldn't any such code, embodying implicit risk and benefit factors (how determined in a given state of knowledge), also tend strongly to preserve it (encrusted with authority)? What would be the likely competence of such agencies (supposing them not to be largely controlled by clinicians) in exercising independent judgment and weighing potential risks and benefits of possible new diagnostic or therapeutic techniques in relation to various kinds of patients in the formulation, interpretation, and modification of such a code? Or in the conception of such new techniques? Answers to questions like these would lend little support to any prima facie merit in such an approach.

It may be said again that various constraints upon experimentation in clinical medicine, as elsewhere in science, are surely justifiable. Many are already at work, and further ones might reasonably be considered needful. But the view that these constraints should be sweepingly enlarged and strengthened, buttressed by the erroneous belief that clinicians engage in no more than applications of rote knowledge, needs tempering with recognition of what is seen as a main point of emphasis: modern clinical medicine is in ordinary and important respects an inherently experimental science. Innovative but also fallible, its activities unavoidably create some human risks while seeking to diminish larger risks. On balance, with an eye to its record and present condition, clinical medicine is a science worthy of nurture and respect.

Point: For several decades after World War II, and issue of the Nuremberg Code (1967) and the Declaration of Helsinki (1966), clinicians in this country (and most other western nations) have had legality in human experimentation. This pillar for advance of medical science comes with strict regulations: Every study involving human beings requires a protocol (detailed description of the entire study), which must be reviewed and passed by an institutional board of experts and lay persons ("IRB"), along with departmental and often sub-committees. Studies are designed for minimal risk and discomfort while obtaining important new medical knowledge.[9] Let this be so.

Medical Algorithms

Clinical interest in diagnostic algorithms has been around for several decades, exemplified as the "decision tree" and "discrimination net" models illustrated in chapter 2. Similar models continue to be proposed in medical literature, but for the most part these models have shown important weaknesses. In his book, Dr. Groopman writes, "Clinical algorithms can be useful for run-of-the-mill diagnoses and treatment—distinguishing strep throat from viral pharyngitis, for example. But they quickly fall apart when a doctor needs to think outside their boxes, when symptoms are big, or multiple and confusing, or when test results are inexact."[10] What are these weaknesses?

Dr. Groopman[11] has the right gist in his quotation above, mostly in the second statement. Even here, however, the phrase "when a doctor needs to think outside their boxes" implies the algorithm is inadequate. The remainder of this statement, "when symptoms are big, or multiple or confusing, or when test results are inexact," strongly suggests the doctor's thinking is analytical, the kind of clinical reasoning dealt thematically within this book.

The first part of Dr. Groopman's quotation, including "distinguishing strep throat from viral pharyngitis," has even more problems. Whatever their size, algorithms work from multiple nexuses connecting (or ending) various pathways. They are quite like a road map, pathways and nexuses being revisable. Unlike roadmaps, reliably taking you to a destination, algorithms are much less dependable. Their weaknesses are multifold, as illustrated in Dr. Groopman's example.

The first weakness is that the likeness of an algorithm to a road map is mostly illusory. Binary turns in towns on a road map are dependable; binary turns (yes or no) at every nexus touched in a working algorithm are less dependable. The uncertainty, probabilities, and complexity in clinical reasoning have wrought the failure of many algorithms in medical diagnosis. Yet, it is not alone that binary nexuses create these problems: they are joined by the pathways.

Note that such pathways may be interpreted as causal or statistical connections, or neither. Either way they may be delinquent in linking signals among nexuses within the format. Along with the binary issues, this metaphor mainly comes down to temporal patterns. An early sign of disease, for example a fever, without any other manifestations, would likely change a good deal over hours and days. Unlike an algorithm, the clinician's knowledge of science, context, and the patient's temporal changes endow her/his superiority.

Algorithms have another serious weakness; they commonly ignore the principle of including all available evidence. Even a small fleeting symptom or sign can warn of high risk to the patient. Algorithms tend to be built for speed, not nuances or patient utilities.

Algorithms can be used in computers, and can also be used by clinicians.[12-16] Accordingly, the term "algorithmic" has been linked with other terms, including "intuitive," "automatic," and "heuristic" (here "short cut"), dealing with quick mind grasp on a medical situation, more or less indicative of a diagnosis. In the compass of fuzzy theory,[17] this group of terms, including algorithmic, can be construed as versions of the traditional clinical term "pattern recognition." Differences between these terms, practical or semantic, these may be charged to their origins and uses among different disciplines, notably psychology and medicine. Clinicians are most familiar with pattern recognition; when this occurs it provides a quick mind set in a direction of a likely diagnosis. Nowadays, however, the clinician would call for tests to further define and confirm the diagnosis, as discussed earlier (chapter 4). The hypotheses-inferential model readily accommodates these procedures.

Medical Ethics

Ethics in medicine is another topic with scope beyond this book. Nonetheless, this subject brings up issues that call for comment.

One issue raises the question, are the terms "ethics" and "morals" identical? It is true that these terms are commonly used interchangeably. Thus, T. Beauchamp and J. Childress write, "Our claim is merely that we draw from the common morality to formulate the principles of biomedical ethics in our book."[18]

Following Beauchamp and Childress, the "up-down" and "down-up" models convey a kind of vertical metaphor. Coupled with a Venn diagram, it is quite simple to display an area within or overlapping circles (as they share at least some content).[19] Supposing both models have some differing features, the down-up model may be of more importance in clinical diagnosis. This might be expected due to more usage of common folk morality, compared to more likely austere ethical precepts, depending on time, place, and people. Both models, however, brings this important element, mostly embedded in tacit knowledge, to the clinician's reasoning through the diagnostic process.[20-21] The goal of the patient's best interest, highly situational and including ethics and morals, demands appropriate clinical judgement. Most clinicians try to do this for every patient—given time, as will be discussed soon. This will extend beyond ethics and morality, including other personal attributes potentially bearing on medical diagnosis. Note in this context, features of ethics and morality belong to the patient.

Medical Values and Utilities

Some observers might question a place for ethics and morality in medical science, given that these features are mostly absent among other sciences—e.g., physical sciences. Nonetheless, other sciences (e.g., psychology) include more or less such attributes as in medical science. Along with ethics and morality, what beliefs and behaviors would fit in this category? How are they discovered in patients? Are they objective or subjective? Are they important? How do values and utilities differ? Do they affect treatment as well as diagnosis? A few brief comments follow.

Patient beliefs and behavior: It is fair to say that no two human persons are identical. One might allow that a scant few "identical" twins are indeed identical, as found by weight and morphology, etc. Despite near perfect similarity at some births, life histories will not be identical, even in utero (different fingerprints), at delivery, and first born. As time goes by, identical twins will be subject to different experiences, e.g., injuries, diseases, social encounters and activities. Even in early childhood, each twin has her/his own medical history. Ordinary siblings, step-siblings, first cousins, second and third cousins, etc., all have differing medical histories. Common unrelated persons have many differences, including medical histories. Yet two persons may have some common genetic traits in immune tolerance, allowing organ transplantation. Ethics and morality are clearly involved in such medical decisions. In fact, these cardinal rules are involved in every clinical judgment.

Values and Utilities: These two terms are closely associated, much like morals and ethics. They are also associated with subjective and objective perspectives. The patient's pain is subjective; her/his smile with thanks to the observing clinician, the objective signs of relief. But were the signs true, or not? Was the "smile" only forced, the "thanks" for trying? The experienced clinician will pursue the examination of the patient until tentatively satisfied. Throughout this process, the clinician will allow a suspicious finding, perhaps subtle, to steer more detailed testing.[22] "Tentatively satisfied" means a simple diagnosis [e.g., laceration on the arm] or more complex cases involving more exams and technical testing from a list of differential diagnoses. Previously discussed, this process has ranks of importance for the clinician to sort out.

On a list of diagnostic hypotheses, each will have a rough probability of being correct. In testing, there will be juggling of these probabilities from start to finish, as evidence mounts. In the usual absence of a pathognomonic disease, the diagnostic hypothesis with the highest probability is commonly favored, perhaps like some games. Unlike games, experienced clinicians know that it is the diagnostic hypothesis with the greatest risk that should be tested first[21]—given the risk has not already been disconfirmed by other testing, within temporal efficacy, etc. The clinician must use judgment in dealing with situational (mitigating or amplifying) factors of risk, including the patient's condition and wishes. Note also that essentially all of the diagnostic hypotheses have their own risks, for the clinician to weigh among others, depending on the condition and wishes of the patient.

Dealing with values and utilities, a renowned philosopher of science, Ian Hacking, writes, "Decisions need more than probability."[22] He goes on to describe "utiles" such: "The expected value of an act is the sum of the products (utilities x probabilities)"[23] (emphasis original), and further writes, "The expected value rule does not factor in such attitudes as risk aversion..."[24] (emphasis mine). The clinician would ordinarily deal with a patient's "risk aversion" (not uncommon), among many other "attitudes." Professor Hacking is to be credited for his thorough and insightful work.

Evidence-Based Medicine

Evidence-based medicine (EBM) was founded by G. Guyatt, Professor of Epidemiology at McMaster University in Hamilton, Ontario, in 1991.[25] Many books and articles following on this subject attest to its interest among clinicians, hospitals, governments, and others. What kind of approach to patients is this?

It is a methodological model. It stands upon a foundation of statistics, dismissing most traditional medical knowledge, especially theory.[26-29] This maneuver is used to rid the model of bias (cf. below) as much as possible.[30] Additionally, the maneuver is viewed by some as bringing other benefits, including simplification and treatment of patients. Note that this model is in use for both diagnosis and treatment, and this discussion will center on clinical diagnosis, with perhaps just a bit of treatment. It will also offer some comparisons of EBM with the hypotheses-inferential (H-I) model as presented in previous chapters.

Model Structures

Example One

<u>H-I</u>: Most clinicians are familiar with the traditional (professional) diagnostic model, she/he beginning with the patient's history and physical examination. A simple observable finding, an ordinary skin laceration, is diagnosed and treated. If there are no other complaints or manifestations of illness, the patient may be released, or the clinician may extend the history, ask again if the patient fell or was abused, etc., before other procedures are indicated, if needed, and then the patient released.

Given the patient dealt with above, a simple skin laceration, the EBM diagnosis and treatment are likely to be similar. The four steps are interesting and will be discussed. First, however, both models will be tested again, now dealing with a couple of more complex patients.

Example Two

<u>H-I</u>: Going back (Chapter 5) to a discussion of a similar gentleman with painful throat and fever for two days. This man complains that some of his family have recently had the flu, about a week ago, and he must have caught the illness. He feels sick all over, with coughing and muscle and joint aching, and has some dizziness and headache. He feels a little short of breath. He lately has trouble with urination and noticed skimpy volume since getting sick, but also has nausea and little appetite for food and fluids. His exam showed temperature of 101 degrees, borderline hypertension, pulse 95/minute, heart sounds normal, breathing 20/minute, chest auscultation of slight basal rales, no definite pitting around the ankles, prostate normal, and moderate

pharyngitis. He adds that he had an illness a few months ago, just a sore throat and fever. He had no doctor visits then or since. He has at times wondered if his heart is weak, but he has no known episodes or heart tests. An initial RADT test for Strep A is negative. He insists he has the flu and wants to go home. He says he needs a drink, but denies having too much. Given her/his questions and exam, the clinician is unsure of this. His dehydration was treated. What more may the clinician do?

H-I: The clinician continues the interview and exam as she/he develops a list of differential diagnoses, likely to include systemic viral illness, Strep A pharyngitis, urinary infection, pneumonia, dehydration (treated), concern of weak heart, and possible alcohol abuse. The clinician works up all of these possible diagnoses by testing their consequent evidence (chapter 6). Laboratory tests likely include Strep A RADT test, CBC, liver function, and urinalysis and culture. Other procedures include chest x-ray, ECG, and consultation of cardiologist (if available). These procedures revealed minor abnormalities. The cardiologist scheduled a follow-up examination, but the patient did not show up.

EBM: The clinician uses a few minutes to compare this patient's illness to patients with a pharyngitis, fever, and body aches. He is dehydrated and has been given appropriate IV fluids. RADT was negative. No antibiotic was given. Despite a rule of statistical likelihood ratio in the USA, given the high specificity of RADT,[31] a throat culture was not obtained. Like above, the cardiologist scheduled a follow-up examination, but the patient did not show up.

Example Three

<u>H-I</u>: To her/his surprise, the clinician found the patient discussed above (example two) in her/his exam room about ten years later. The patient had been brought to the emergency room with an obvious new fracture of his distal right tibia, judged likely fibula also. He was groggy and could barely speak. He was walking on a sidewalk when he blacked out and fell. He came in an ambulance. The clinician noted moderate weakness in the left extremities, suspicious of a stroke. The clinician also noted mild jaundice, firm liver, enlarged spleen, ascites, telangiectasia, edema to the knees from ankles and feet, blood pressure normal, erratic pulse at 115/minute, temperature 99.5, diastolic heart murmur, marked lung rales, shortness of breath, and slight productive cough. The patient states he is in pain about his leg fracture. He admits to smoking forty pack years. He also mentioned his numerous allergies to pills, noticed for a few years, including some pain pills. Excitedly, trying to raise his voice, he objects to treatment with any blood products. The radiologist arrives to exam the patient, and to discuss the likely stroke and fracture.

About this time, some initial tests are underway, such as ECG, MR imaging of the brain, lab tests, chest x-ray, and perhaps more. Fortunately for our purposes, we don't need the entire story, but what follows are essential: Given the patient's history and physical examination, the clinician lists an initial group of differential-diagnoses. Generally, this will include all organ systems which can have effects on others.[31] Such cause and effect relationships in "co-morbidities" are dealt with in clinical knowledge and diagnostic reasoning. Note that most of these examples work as cover for more detailed hypotheses (e.g., where and type of fracture, stroke, etc.). Important causal nexuses usually claim the term "diagnosis," depending on current medical language.

A tentative and partial <u>differential-diagnosis</u> for this example:

1. Stroke, right hemisphere, acute
2. Pulmonary insufficiency (Oxygen therapy)
3. Mitral stenosis, indeterminate etiology
4. Atrial fibrillation
5. Fracture of the distal right tibia, trauma, acute
6. Fracture of the right fibula, trauma, acute
7. Pulmonary hypertension
8. Right ventricular failure
9. Hepatic cirrhosis
10. Splenomegaly/Hypersplenism
11. COPD
12. Others: milling in the clinician's reasoning, e.g., nature of the stroke, infections (heart, liver, lung, kidney), alcohol abuse/withdrawal, ethics, patient wants, etc.

Mind that these preliminary hypotheses rest on the clinician's history and examination of the patient. Commonly, a good deal of new evidence would later be added from testing (laboratory, imaging, functions, interviews,[32] etc.). Most of these tests are guided by the list of hypotheses, used like evidential tools to select confirmatory hypotheses/diseases. Generally, neutral, inconsistent, or disconfirmatory hypotheses/diagnoses are likely to be set aside (Chapter 6). Mind also the cardinal principle in the H-I model that <u>all relevant and available evidence</u> must be used until the clinician's judgements are satisfied. Particularly, hypotheses/diseases with even very low (yet real) probability, but very high risk to the patient, or others, should always be guarded. Hence, through the diagnostic process, the list of differential-diagnoses remains flexible, depending on the patient's condition and best care.

EBM: The clinician had also seen the patient about ten years ago. What she/he does depends on age and experience: (I) younger and always looks to EBM, and (2) any age but mostly experience and traditional causal reasoning, little use of EBM. Perhaps the latter would follow the work-up diagnoses and treatment similarly to the clinicians described above (H-I). However, the clinician (I) has problems getting on track with the patients such as above, examples 2 and 3, concerning all the steps. Brief comments will accompany each step.

Step1: "Define a clinical question and its four components: Patient, intervention, comparison and outcome."[33]

Comment: The five categories in this sentence (including "clinical question") have wide scope, but short of details. The four components in this statement are held high, somewhat like enshrined in the mnemonic, "PICO." This can be found in EBM literature in discussion of Step1, e.g., "EBM courses are doctrinaire in their approach and require participants to follow a set method to EBM problems."[34]

Step2: "Find the evidence that will help answer the question. PubMed Clinical Queries is an efficient database to accomplish this step."[35]

Comment: An experienced and knowledgeable clinician knows when to seek new information involving a patient, whether consultation with another colleague, or looking into reference literature like PubMed. Remember too that clinicians are mandated to attend medical lectures, reviews and discussions (at least 75 hours / 3 years in USA), and intermittent testing of nearly all clinicians in their specialties.

Step3: "Assess whether this evidence is valid and important. A quick review of the methods and results section will help to answer these two questions."[36]

Comment 1: The authors offer an example of bias: "Some troponin studies assess troponin results in predicting final discharge/diagnosis/management/outcome, forgetting that if the troponin was revealed to the clinician during admission, it will have inevitably affected diagnosis, management and outcome."[37] This early surprise of having relevant and important evidence should help both the clinician and patient. The experienced clinician assimilates changes in the patient along with few or many test results throughout the diagnostic process, and is skilled to do so. The proposal above describing requirements for the reference standard brings up again the shrine of EBM. (Cf. bias below).

Comment 2: The author's question, "Was the diagnostic test evaluated in an appropriate population of patients comparable to the patient of interest?" It should be clear if the patient group assessed was similar in age, sex, race, location (inpatient, outpatient, emergency department, primary care) and presenting symptoms to the patient of interest. Many studies of diagnostic tests use clearly healthy vs. clearly diseased patients for their assessments, giving over-optimistic assessments of the performance characteristics, "and is the cause of many of the differences in reported sensitivity and specificity figures found in the literature."[38]

This is no doubt true and opens the issue of fitting a particular patient (of interest) to an appropriate reference standard, but how many and which patients fit into this methodological model? Looking back to Example Three, the H-I model works well, whereas EBM easily stumbles. Why? Because the patient has many and complex conditions and co-morbidities, as well as ethical personal wishes. Not only are there problems with diagnosis, but also EBM guidelines for treatment of patients with co-morbidities, especially common among older patients.

<u>Step4</u>: "Apply the evidence to the patient. This step includes: assessing whether the test can be used; determining if it will help the patient; finding whether the study patients are similar to the patient in question; determining a pretest probability; and deciding if the test will change one's management of the patient."[39]

Comment 1: "Apply the evidence to the patient."[40] This sentence itself carries a range of meaning and significance for the patient, so back to our categories of diseases. An ordinary skin laceration (Example 1) should not in general be difficult for diagnosis, if needed details being provided by the surgeon. Note that some observable signs and symptoms can connect with systemic disease (e.g., scleroderma, lupus, etc.), or signs like jaundice and telangiectasia. These can be seen as "complex," and as parts of one disease. Manifestations in such an example—depending on timing and other variables, including typicality—may fit a certain pattern for use of EBM. Unlike this, however, the patient with two or more diseases is likely to be more complicated, due to abnormal causes and effects between organ systems, as well as a mix of manifestations. This will be discussed again in a following segment.

Comment 2/3: "This step includes: assessing whether the test can be used; determining if it will help the patient."[41] This coupling may help to clarify the situation of the test. The first part ("whether the test can be used") suggests several meanings, e.g., risk (many kinds); machine is out of order (MR is down, CT is safe and useful), scheduling (should be fixable), patient concerns (discussion with clinician), cost, etc. Note that some risks are more significant than others are and may be recognized as dominant on this list. This set aside, there may at times be a tendency, or even block, to avoid costs of certain tests. This would largely stem from complicated USA insurance companies and/or medical management organizations. This too aside, the clinician herself/himself in such a test situation will be "determining if it will help the patient."[42] At this point, how firm—if at all—is the patient's diagnosis? Would the test results surprisingly suggest a different diagnosis? Whatever the diagnosis, would the test results mainly affect the patient's values or quality of life?

Comment 4: "Finding whether the study patients are similar to the patient in question."[43] This question again brings vagaries. What is meant by "similar"? Think of a list of terms, starting with just medical terms. Then there should be general terms, like "values"[44] and about the question in "whether"—yes or no?" To be easily satisfied with a short list of terms, and the answer "yes," is to rely on assumptions and biases.[45,46] The latter is not all bad, for all humans have biases (cf. below). Science has a reputation for un-biasing. Science, however, argues assumptions in randomized clinical trials, such that the more alike the study patients, if generalized, the less likely to be similar to a new patient. Is Step 4 in EBM truly scientific? Ethical?

Comment 5: "Determining the pretest probability."[47] This question also has difficulties, affecting both H-I and EBM models. For both, pretest probability (PP) can seem simple, e.g., in a game of coin tossing and counting heads and tails, say ten tosses. Mr. A bets more counts on heads, Mr. B takes tails. Heads wins with seven, tails gets three. They continue, this time to a hundred tosses. Tails show up lower than 50%. Mr. B. felt justified in results of objective (frequency) probabilities, but he had not recognized the coin. He pondered if the coin was fair or not—a step into subjective probability.

The simple point of this little story should illustrate the concept and daily range of human uncertainty. Major points should include the complimentary mix of objective and subjective models of probability[48] and their uses in clinical reasoning (Chapter 5). The effort in the EBM model in dealing with the pretest probability is similar to certain features of the H-I model. When needed in either model, review of pertinent medical literature can provide information. To my knowledge, however, such information can fail to be available, current, detailed, unusual cases, etc. The clinician with scientific medical knowledge and experience, along with pertinent literature or consulting colleagues, if needed, can best manage such situations. She/he will fit pretest probabilities, combining objective and subjective probabilities, as most suitable, when formulating the list of differential diagnoses.

Comment 6: "And deciding if the test will change one's management of the patient." This rule will leave us with some ambiguity. Mainly, it will depend on the timing of this decision in the context of other decisions. A few of these will be noted.

First: Deciding on the test must be done, if at all, after firm diagnosis and management plan. This can be problematic, whenever other potential diagnoses may be affected by the test, especially those with significant risk.

Second: A test may provide information not helpful to the clinician's management plan, but still be beneficial to the patient. For example, patients have been affected by mild brain injury, including concussion, for essentially all time. Despite recent societal awakening, patients with such injuries have been slow to receive medical diagnosis and treatment.

Third: One could say that today's record of a patient's health care now will be much of the groundwork for her/his future health care.

Fourth: It is true that medical tests can be expensive. Nonetheless, many common tests are not so expensive. For example, a medical clinic in suburban Minneapolis charges only $35 for a common test, the Complete Blood Counts (CBC; a total of ten blood tests). In a hospital, a CBC costs $69, and a three-view chest x-ray costs $123.

Missed diagnoses also tend to be expensive. The knowledgeable and experienced clinician may prefer judgement, rather than mandate, throughout and after the patient's diagnostic process.

H-I and EBM Medical Diagnosis Models: Special Aspects

Connecting evidence with diagnosis

Remarkably, ICD-10 has classified at least 12,000 medical diagnoses (diseases, disorders, conditions, etc.) and many more at this time. These are from around the world, along with those indigenous in the United States. Even if only the latter, despite knowing otherwise, it would amount to a large group. Additional to this is the matter of comorbidities, another group of potential patients with either several singular codes or sometimes combinations of coded diagnoses. Briefly, how do H-I and EBM clinicians work in these circumstances? As shown in this book, the H-I clinician will gather initial relevant evidence from the patient's history and examination, then creates a list of reasonably probable diagnoses, the latter being the cause(s) of the patient's unwanted manifestations, then a process of such cycles until the clinician is satisfied that the riddles are adequately answered. This being a process, when needed the good clinician keeps an eye and ear to be sure.

The parallel process of EBM depends in large part on a deluge of clinical trial studies, with a fair bit of ambiguity. The model stipulates many rules for the clinician to follow, of which the reference standard is generally dominant. The latter (at times called the "question") denotes a certain—or uncertain—statistical group (cohort) that appears to have disease manifestations similar to those of the patient of interest. The clinician searches for the correct (or best) comparable group of studies. At this point, notice that the clinician should have good medical knowledge and experience to be able to get this far, even with available literature. Next, the clinician obtains new relevant evidence—if needed, testing. Test results can confirm or disconfirm, and may call for a different group (or groups) of studies. How does this differ from the H-I model? Again, we go to levels of complexity, as described in examples 1-3.

Level One: Fortunately, there are many relatively simple diagnoses in medicine. Some in this category are simply observable, such as sun burn, or benign skin laceration. Not all skin lesions are simple, however, needing dermatology, perhaps biopsy and surgery. On the other hand, some non-observable diagnoses can be simple, sometimes such as a dislocated shoulder, or at times cardiac rhythms. Both EBM and H-I models should work in these contexts, but with H-I generally having a larger scope, brought up in the differential list.

Level Two: It might suffice to say that this position hovers quietly about midway between the two ends. We know that diagnoses gain complexity with increasing co-morbidities, but this is not all, as other factors contribute. In particular, causal effects between organ systems affect their functions. Subordinate patho-physiology and mechanisms can affect other, at times unusual, organ systems. Thus, another factor in such conditions would involve the clinician, she/he being knowledgeable and understanding of scientific processes affecting the patient. Without these conditions, how easily (accurately, thoroughly) might the clinician connect the evidence to a cohort?

Level Three: This is the opposite end of simple, merging into complex and difficult diseases and co-morbidities, and beyond to new knowledge, causes and effects for an old disease (e.g., heliocobacter pylori), or causes and effects for new diseases (influenza, HIV, Ebola, etc.). Causes and effects from genetic mutations, and other faults, also belong in this category.[50]

I don't have the numbers, but it seems that there are many more diseases (including conditions, disorders, etc.) than their cumulative signs and symptoms (manifestations), with interview and physical examination but without evidence by other testing.[51] Unlike the H-I model, the EBM clinician is ruled to avoid such testing before choosing a reference standard, boosting the EBM clinician's challenge with a patient's complex diagnoses. Having a reference standard settled, testing can then be done, if deemed needed, for evidence to support or diminish the diagnosis. If this fails, the first diagnosis is ruled out, and another diagnosis is tried.[52] Unlike the EBM model, the H-I clinician builds a list of reasonable diagnostic hypotheses, whether simple or complex, the contending probabilities shift with confirmatory, or disconfirmatory, test results. The clinician deals with knowledge of patho-physiology, along with objective and/or subjective probabilities, in diagnostic reasoning. As discussed above, utilities in hypotheses with low probability but risk to the patient (or others) would generally be ruled out (or in) on the clinician's judgment.

Patterns of Recognition

As mentioned above, few signs and symptoms can be misleading. Busy clinicians may at times welcome short cuts[53] when working with patient diagnoses. A large part of such short cuts deals with simple diagnoses, and with epidemics. For example, cerebral spinal fluid leaking through the nose might be mistaken to a common cold. Unfortunately, these situations may lend cause to missed diagnoses. Any clinician could make such mistakes, but H-I differential lists should help avoid it.

Another usage of "pattern recognition" deals with more complex and chronic diseases. Three of these conditions have involved the endocrine systems for several decades: acromegaly, Cushing's syndrome, and hyperthyroidism. All of these have progressed in medical science, and some new names. On a first meeting with such a patient, however, the clinician might abruptly bring to mind a diagnosis, by way of mental short cuts or pattern recognition, but the meaning of the diagnosis is not the same as a decade or two, or perhaps a year ago. It has changed because science has found new or refined medical knowledge of these diseases. For example, hyperthyroidism and its effects on the patient (at times eyes, etc.) has been known for nearly two centuries. Following Caleb Parry's observations on thyroid disease in the late eighteenth century, the Irish surgeon Robert J. Graves (Dublin, 1796-1853) hypothesized a connection between goiter and exophthalmos. He published his new thyroid disease in 1835, called with his name, Graves, to this day.[54] A second disease connected with hyperthyroidism was discovered by Dr. Henry Stanley Plummer (1874-1936).[55,56] A professor at the Mayo Clinic, Dr. Plummer found that thyroid nodules could release excessive amounts of hormone, causing the thyroid to become toxic. An inventive physician, among other contributions, Dr. Plummer made this discovery in 1913 and the disease "toxic multinodular goiter" has been called by his name since. Several contemporary diseases of hyperthyroidism include singular over-functioning nodule (sometimes also called "Plummer," or just "hot nodule"), excess stimulation of the thyroid by another hormone (TSH) from the pituitary gland, too much iodine, thyroiditis (inflammation), and excess exogenous thyroid hormone. Clearly, the meaning and usage of "pattern recognition" has changed in dealing with hyperthyroidism due to medical science providing discoveries and new knowledge. It is interesting that both Dr. Robert Graves and Dr. Henry Plummer began their professional medical careers in private practice. Many clinicians continue today to offer an important scientific role between academia and private practice. Will EBM support this among clinicians?[57] In regard to pattern recognition, this works like a platform for short cuts, but not very well, simply because there are not many of them that clinicians can rely upon.

Scientific Medicine and Some Recent History

Looking back to two general classifiers in medical science, one being causal, and the other being correlation (Chapter 2), this section will again briefly aim for the division of these terms. Most everyone knows about causes and correlations, but their differences can be important in medical science.

A simple causal event, as generally understood, is an antecedent phenomenon (one or more) to one or more of its subsequent effects. An example would include a billiard ball moving straight on to hit a second but unmoving billiard ball. What will happen? Most people will know the first ball will collide and stop, and the second ball begins rolling. People will know this, even if not familiar with billiard balls. Why won't footballs work? This common knowledge grows naturally from empiric experience. In fact, such empiric generalizations obey— even constitute—natural laws. Our simple system of billiard balls, with more details, is proper within the realm of physics. It happens that the laws of (macro) physics also work in medical science (see an example by Dr. Malcolm Potts on "Parachute approach to evidence based medicine").[58] Other sciences also play a role in medical science (chemistry, psychology, pharmaceuticals, etc.). Nonetheless, medical science stands and works overwhelmingly in its own domains, the largest and most important being clinical diagnosis and treatment of patients and their potential myriad diseases, disorders, injuries, etc. Does this actually affect a family clinician? Surely so.

Using the H-I model, medical science uses powerful methods, analogous with other sciences. For our purposes, the investigation of cause and effect linkages of (macro) empiric phenomena is just such a method. These causal linkages allow us to explain and predict events, whether by natural laws or tendency laws, by certainty or probabilistic, as previously discussed (Chapter 4).

Thinking again about the thyroid, Dr. Robert Graves noticed the correlation between goiters (hyperthyroidism) and exophthalmos in about 1835. I have no knowledge that Dr. Graves, a surgeon, tried surgery on a goiter, but other surgeons did so during the mid and late nineteenth century.[59] Despite the moderate frequency of exophthalmos among patients with goiters,[60] it seems this association came to be seen as causal linkage. It is now believed that an immune disease causes both of the thyroid and eye diseases. As above, there is now known several other causes for clinical hyperthyroidism.

We are at a couple of other points. The thyroid gland and conjoining systems (pituitary, hormones, receptors, infections, human behavior), create an array of scientific causes and effects. Every empiric generalization describing one of these connections, even if firmly established (held as knowledge), belongs in the category of scientific theory. Remember Isaac Newton (English physicist, 1643-1727), the falling apple(s), and the orbit of the moon around the earth, all due to gravity. Newton's theories were heraldic at his time, and remain useful still, but with less refinement and accuracy compared with the newer theory of general relativity founded by Albert Einstein (German/American, 1879-1955). Should we now believe theory in physics (chemistry, etc.) is just about completed? Does anyone have answers to the dark mass/energy? After several decades of work, the Higgs boson was recently identified. Neutrinos, extremely small particles (hard to catch), coming in huge numbers from the sun, flying through human beings essentially all of the time, with probable miniscule interaction.[61] There are other theories in basic sciences that are not well established or not have useful causal linkages with medical science. More important, however, there are many such causal linkages going back at least to the time of Galileo (Italian,

1564–1642).[62,63] For our purposes, skip time and growing science in the interim, looking again in the late nineteenth century, when two startling discoveries came on stage: X-rays and radioactivity. X-rays came first, by Wilhelm C. Rontgen (German physicist, 1845-1923), discovered while experimenting with charged vacuum tubes, in 1895. Remarkably, Henri Becquerel (French physicist, 1852-1908) and Marie Curie (Polish physicist and chemist, 1867-1934) worked together in discovering elements emitting radioactivity, in 1896. All three of these scientists were awarded with Nobel Prizes, Rontgen (Physics, 1901), Becquerel (Physics, 1903), and Mme. Curie (Physics, 1903). A towering scientist, including her discoveries of radioactive elements (thorium, polonium, radium), she received a second Nobel award in Chemistry (1911). Mme. Curie is said to have helped with medical uses of x-rays during World War I.[64]

These three scientists' work in a few years, about a century ago, changed the world of scientific medicine. Mme Curie called X-rays and their use in medicine the field of "radiology." She also used the word "radio" similarly for the term "radioactivity." The benefits and hazards of radioactive exposure were not well understood at that time. Unfortunately, Mme Curie herself sickened and died in 1934 of aplasia anemia.[64] Nonetheless, knowledge of uses of radioactive elements in medical diagnosis and treatment grew, and surged in mid-twentieth century with the innovation of nuclear medicine, continuing today with many new types of radioactive materials (Chapter 1). This progress is a powerful example of conjoining parts of physics and medical science, their reward not just to the scientist or science alone, but to benefit all humanity.

My understanding is that EBM has little or no use for theory: statistics only—or just maybe? My view on this is "just maybe." Suppose advocates of EBM attempt to shutter contemporary medical knowledge completely. This would not be workable, even by pattern recognition. Suppose advocates of EBM would accept all such medical knowledge and its uses. This would not be seen as EBM. It seems then that EBM clinicians must allow some uses of usual (their) medical knowledge, as needed. Like the story above, scientific knowledge, including medical science, is permeated with theory (Chapter 1). This applies also to the science within EBM. The methodology of EBM calls for a strict framework of procedures, typically paring or discarding parts of medical knowledge. This parting should include theory (medical generalizations) and other medical knowledge left out in favor of new statistics (Chapter 9). Some may reply that EBM clinicians must (if possible) use fresh medical knowledge, as can be found in digital literature, like PubMed and others. Fortunately, all clinicians in our country and other countries should have access to similar information. Unfortunately, however, EBM clinicians working with a rigid methodological framework, kept away from large parts of commonly used medical knowledge, it would be unsurprising that she/he have to struggle with moderate or complex diseased patients. Nor is it good for these patients, and so for others, given problems in triage.

Scientific Medicine and its Future

The H-I model emphasizes the common medical knowledge and its full usage by learned and experienced clinicians. The growth of medical knowledge during recent decades has prompted some clinicians for both common and specialized medical knowledge, along with experience to be categorized as experts. It is important that such clinicians may confer with colleagues, if needed, for information from other parts of medical knowledge—or turn to digital literature (simplified, commonly binary, often a few years old, inconsistencies…). Instead, from time to time, clinicians may come upon a curiosity, a variant, or possibly new condition or disease. The mandatory medical conferences draw typical back and forth discussions, usually after lectures, but also at round table meetings. Remarkably, general clinicians have much to hear, and much to say. I will claim again that there is no fixed line or divide between physicians—laboratory research, teaching, full time care of patients, all are professional and clinicians. This has been quite similar throughout medical history. Like other sciences, this methodology has brought the knowledge and wonders to modern medicine—and many wonders yet to come, if the proven methodology is not broken down. Has this begun to happen, along with other trends, in places where large scale EBM rules? Dr. Desmond J. Sheridan recently wrote the book, "Evidence-Based Medicine: Best Practice or Restrictive Dogma." Despite his many softeners, he is critical of the wide sweep of recent UK methods failing in making progress in clinical science.[65] His words:

"The decline in clinical science in recent decades has been a major contributing factor to our failure to adapt advances in science for the benefit of patients, now known as the translation gap. An even more serious consequence is our failure even to consider the possibilities that original science can bring to such problems as antimicrobial resistance, preferring instead to focus on making the best of what we have now. This reversal of the great strides made in the early 20th century to introduce science into clinical settings ..., and its retreat back to the laboratory is surely one of the great tragedies to befall medicine in the UK in recent decades. Commitment to science and new knowledge are values intrinsic to medicine because they are essential to maintaining to progress and standards of excellence and the decline of recent decades has been harmful to both. Sooner or later the failures which these have caused will demand a rethink as they did at the beginning of the 20th century."[66]

Issues and comments

Dr. Sheridan brings up several major issues in his concise and fertile paragraph above.[66] It may be useful to read it in pieces, with some comments for our purposes.

(1)   "The decline in clinical science in recent decades has been a major contributing factor to our failure to adapt advances in science for the benefit of patients, now known as the translation gap."

        Comment: Dr. Sheridan writes primarily on conditions in UK, where EBM seems abundant. Given its doctrinaire form and use, however, it should have similar effects in other countries, including USA. See also comments (2) and (3).

(2)   "An even more serious consequence is our failure even to consider the possibilities that original science can bring to such problems as antimicrobial resistance, preferring instead to focus on making the best of what we have now."

        Comment: An army of professional clinicians in the field communicating with research clinicians could recognize and assist in new and better patient care.

(3)   "This reversal of the great strides made in the early 20th century to introduce science into clinical settings…"

        Comment: Today's medical knowledge continues to owe scientific methods in clinical medicine, especially in the last century. This could be called a paradigm.

(4)   "…and its retreat back to the laboratory is surely one of the great tragedies to befall medicine in the UK in recent decades."

Comment: See comment in (1).

(5)   "Commitment to science and new knowledge are values
       intrinsic to medicine because they are essential to maintain-
       ing progress and standards of excellence and the decline of
       recent decades has been harmful to both."

Comment: The beginning of this piece claims the importance of science in medicine, acknowledged by many others, including one's first article.[67] The last statement, including "decline," brings to mind Professor Thomas Kuhn (b.1922 – d.1996, Harvard), creator of the term "paradigm." Well off the progress of medical science in the twentieth century, Kuhn wrote of medicine thus: "Established crafts like medicine, calendar making and metallurgy."[68] Kuhn was not a physician, and his understanding of modern medical science can be overlooked, given his many other contributions. Nonetheless, who today would aim medical science for this picture?

(6)   "Sooner or later the failures which these have caused will
       demand a rethink as they did at the beginning of the
       20th century."

Comment: One believes sooner, for benefits to clinicians and patients. Follow the medical maxim: "treat the cause, not only the symptoms."[69]

Bias

Bias is an innate feature of human beings, whether aimed at food, love, power, and so on. It is built into our nature, helping us to keep satisfied and even alive. Humans also have other powerful features, like caring for others, bravery, productivity, etc. An ensemble of such features in an individual human being counts as "character" (see below). My experience with clinicians puts most of them in high tiers of character. Nonetheless, all have some biases.[70] Are there no human activities with fewer biases?

Many would answer "science," yet parts of science continue to be divisive, e.g., physics (cosmology, dark matter, string theory), and more or less every other science.[71] Science needs to grow. If not, it may over time devolve into a kind of "craft" (Chapter 1). This is not the situation of medical science, now or for many decades and indeed centuries ago. There surely are many challenges to bring new medical knowledge, offer better understanding of causes and mechanisms, and better treatment to allay, or cure, diseases.

One might conjecture an association between decline of a valued science and the rise of its biases, and vice versa, other factors reasonably stable. Generally, we respect and try to maintain or enhance things of value. Is there now such a trend in medical science, up or down? For our answer, we need to look at the biases and status of contemporary medical science. Keep in mind the main purpose of these discussions, sorting out the best methodology in medical diagnosis. The H-I model stands on medical science, logic, probability, and being thorough—patient history, disease complexity, rare diseases, disabilities, values, risk avoidance, common and tacit knowledge, theory, etc.[72-81] The competitor, EBM, may hold some or different items from this list, but essentially stands on a thin platform, depending almost entirely on statistics -- gleaned from hand-picked groups (generalized as "standards"), and depending heavily on pattern recognition, having rid of theory, etc. In practice, the EBM model has been criticized for decline of medical science (in UK, above).[66] Others have more widely faulted EBM, including frequent and weighty biases.[82-84]

On another point, there is the problem of a gap between academic clinicians who work with patients, research, and education (many expert), and clinicians who work mostly or only with patients.[78,81] In fact, many of the latter are also experts. Mandated medical scientific meetings, literature, and periodic testing, along with the clinician's body of medical knowledge and experience, and daily information ("strep throat is going around"), does quite well in covering such a gap. Nonetheless, compared to traditional clinician's professionalism, has there been significant change in their roles, and why? These questions are not wide in my bailiwick, but I have a few thoughts.

EBM: Diagnosis, Outcomes, and Guidelines

These three subjects, or so it seems, have their own EBM methods, being to some extent shared in use. This chapter has compared methodological features of EBM with the traditional "H-I" model of clinical diagnosis. Some other EBM features pertain to categories of patient outcomes and guidelines, with different purposes.

Like diagnostic EBM, outcomes and guidelines depend almost entirely on frequency (objective) statistics, leaving aside causal mechanisms, whether old or new, or scientific or common knowledge. New statistical information is obtained by randomized clinical trials.[85] Despite concept, bias has found human tendencies, especially in publications of such trials.[85-89] An even bigger problem, a formidable barrier, using statistics derived from relatively small and standardized subjects, the results then allowed to expand and generalize to apply to other patients, some or most unfit (non-selected) for the trial. This is called "assumptions," or just "generalizations," well known by EBM advocates and used in the formulations of clinical practice guidelines (CPGs—management and treatment). As with diagnoses, such guidelines are more problematic among patients with unusual or complex diseases.

To expand on the issues of healthcare and costs among older patients, Dr. C. Boyd, et al., published in 2005 a study of chronic diseases among Medicare patients. In their words: "In 1999, 48% of Medicare beneficiaries aged 65 years or older had at least 3 chronic medical conditions and 21% had 5 or more. Healthcare costs for individuals with at least 3 chronic conditions accounted for 89% of Medicare's annual budget." In conclusion, they begin, "This review suggests that adherence to current CPGs in caring for an older person with several comorbidities may have undesirable effects ..." However, physicians who care for older adults with multiple diseases must strike a balance between following CPGs and adjusting recommendations for individual patients' circumstances."[90] An approach to individual patients will be discussed next. First, however, it may be of interest to include a quotation by CL Meinert, thus: "Suppose that the direct cost for generating a person year of follow-up data (2006) is $15,000, producing a direct cost of $450,000 per trial and a total direct cost of 14 billion for the 31,000 trials. The total cost, including indirect costs, will be considerably higher."[91,92] Keep in mind that these trials supply the foundations of the EBM models, using statistics and rules, primarily for CPGs but also for EBM diagnoses in some quarters. Where there is medical literature (USA, Europe, Asia, etc.) most clinicians have access to informative medical statistics. Small studies can be useful quickly (a few weeks, e.g., a wave of infectious disease or food poisoning), with statistics or not, whereas large CPG studies are typically slow in results (a few years).[93] Among "H-I" (traditional) clinicians, subjective probabilities are used when needed for care of patients (Chapter 5).

The Individual Patient

A certain disease/condition

In the field of medical disease the word "binary" is perhaps most important (accounting definitions and boundaries, and not accounting electrons and such) in identifying a certain disease or condition in a given patient. In brief, if a patient has a disease then she/he cannot not have it at the same time, or vice versa.[94] In other words, a certain disease ("D") can be severe or mild, short or lengthy in affliction, residual effects or none, engagement with other certain diseases, etc. These situations are simple, and could be widened by similar elements and details.

The patient

The core amidst all of this discussion is the patient. Let us count the ways she/he may either beguile or show instead her/his uncountable factors, facets, and more. Ordinary human persons begin with unique sets of genes, making them unique. Recall that "identical" twins are not true identical, and NASA has recently shown that environment can modify genes. With time and experience, both single and twin persons will add to their differences, including occurrences of injuries, conditions, and diseases, as for other persons. Uniqueness grows medical knowledge (hence specialties) but is generally constrained by established scientific medical laws and generalizations. Nonetheless, clinicians may at times turn up an unsuspected finding, a puzzling outlier, perhaps an unusual part of a tendency law. If not a researcher, she/he (scientific clinician) would likely discuss with one, as well as other colleagues, typical at medical meetings. This squarely differs from the EBM model wherein communication depends largely on rules and rulers, difficulty with translational gap, and decline in new medical science.[95]

REFERENCES AND FOOTNOTES: CHAPTER 8

1. Cabot, R. C. , Op cit. p. 19
2. Jabs D., American J. of Ophthalmology August 2013, "Approach to the Diagnosis of Yveitides" pp228-236.
3. Bowen J., NEJM Number 23, 2006;355 "Educational Strategies to Promote Clinical Diagnostic Reasoning." pp 2217 – 2225
4. Barrows, H.S., Clinical and Investigative Medicine. Vol 5, No 1. (1982) "The Clinical Reasoning of Randomly Selected Physicians in General Medical Practice." pp 49-55
5. Berghman R., BMJ 2011:343" d5469 "Sir Karl Popper, swans and the general practitioner." pp 1-2
6. Berghman R., and Schouten H. C., Ibid. pp 1-2
7. Feinstein, A., Op cit. ". . . a clinician performs an experiment every time he treats a patient." (Clinical Judgement, p. 14
8. In an autobiographical sketch W. Alvarez, a noted clinical diagnostician and researcher, writes: "There were many clinical questions to which I so much wanted answers that I kept hard at work, with a small notebook continually in my pocket. Today, at seventy-one, I am still eagerly following the clinical studies that fascinated me in 1912, . . . there is a great desire in me to teach others what I have learned. Some people ask me, "What drives you?' . . . I think it is mainly the older hunger for answers to scientific questions, the same hunger which impelled a young boy. . ." ("On Following a Gleam in Science," in Doctors and Patients, ed. N. Fabricant [New York: Grune and Stratton, 1959], p. 112.) Is this attitude less noble here than elsewhere in science?
9. Similar procedures are followed in experiments involving animals.
10. Groopman, J., Op cit., p5
11. Groopman, J., Ibid., p5

12. Croskerry P., Academy Medicine, volume 84, number 8, August 2009. "A universal model of diagnostic reasoning." pp 1022-1028

13. Liu M., J Am Inform Assoc 2012;19:e28-e35 "Algorithmic Predictions of Adverse Drug Reactions" Pe28

14. Stanovitch K., "Distinguishing the reflective algorithmic minds: is it time for tri-partitetheory?" in Evans j., Oxford University Press, "In two minds dual processing and beyond." (2009) pp55-80

15. Norman G., Academic medicine, vol 75, number 10, October Suppl. (2000} "The Epistemology of clinical reasoning: perspectives from philosophy, psychology and neuroscience." (1999} Jack Maatsch Memorial Presentation. pp S127-S133

16. Benner E., The American Journal of Medicine (2008) volume 121 (5A) Overconfidence of a cause of diagnostic error in medicine." pp S2-S23

17. Reyna V., American Psychological Society (2004) volume 13 Number 2 "How people make decisions that involve risk: a dual processes approach." pp60-66

18. Beauchamp T., and Childress J., Oxford University Press (1013, 7th ed.) "Principles of Bioethical Ethics." p.421

19. Beauchamp T., and Childress J., Ibid pp 398-401

20. Henry, S., Theoretical Medicine and Bioethics 26(2006), "Recognizing Tacit Knowledge in Medical Epistemology." pp189-190 and passim.

21. Lanzola G., Artificial Intelligence in medicine 5 (1993)"Inferential knowledge acquisition" p264

22. Hacking I., Op cit., p32

23. Hacking I., Ibid. p100

24. Hacking I., Ibid p105

25. Sheridan D., "Evidence-Based Medicine: Best Practice or Restrictive Dogma" (2016) Imperial College Press, London WC2H 9HE, UK, p15

26. Greenhalgh T., BMJ 2014; 348: g3725 "Evidence based medicine: a movement in crisis?" pp1-13

27. Zakowski L., Clin Med Res, 2004 Feb;2(1): 63-69 "Evidence-based Medicine: Answering Questions of Diagnosis" p1

28. Tannenbaum, S., Academic Medicine volume 74, number seven July, 1999 "Evidence and expertise: the challenge of the outcomes movement to medical professionalism" pp757-759

29. O'Connor P., JAMA, August 10, 2005 – Vol 204' No 06 "Adding Value to Evidence – Based Clinical Guidelines" pp741-743

30. Terms like "cause" occasionally show up in this literature, pointing to relevant tacit knowledge.

31. Bowen, J., NEJM Number 23, 2006' 355:2217 – 2225"Educational Strategies to Promote Clinical Diagnostic Reasoning." p2217

32. Gil C., BMJ volume 337 May 2005pages 1080 – 1083 "Why clinicians are natural Bayesians." p1080

33. Zakowski, L Op cit p63(1/10)

34. Hawkins, R., Clin Biochem Rev., (2005) May 26 (2) "The Evidence Based Medicine Approach to Diagnosis Testing: practicalities and limitations" pp7-18/1-13

35. Zakowski, L Op cit p63(1?10)

36. Zakowski, L ibid

37. Hawkins, R. Op cit pp7-18/1-13

38. Zakowski, L., Op cit p63(1/10), passim

39. Zakowski. L., ibid

40. Zakowski L, ibid

41. Zakowski L, ibid

42. Zakowski L, ibid

43. Zakowski L, ibid

44. O'Connor, P., JAMA August 10, 2005 Volume 294, No 06"Adding Value to Evidence-based Guidelinespp741-743

45. Meinert C., Oxford University Press Inc.,2011 New York, New York "An insider's guide to clinical trials" pp 28 and passim

46. Every-Palmer S., Journal of Evaluation in Clinical Practice, University of Oxford, March 2014, "How evidence-based medicine is failing due to biased trials and selective publications." pp3-15/18

47. Zakowski, L., OP cit p63(1/10)

48. Hacking I., "An Introduction to Probability and Inductive Logic" Cambridge University Press (2001) pp383-390

49. A worker in a medical billing office recently gave me the number of diagnostic codes (ICD-10) totaled approximately 70,000 .

50. Dauger A., American Academy of Pediatrics: Pediatrics 126(6): e1594-e1598 (2010) "Delayed puberty due to a novel mutation in CHD7causing a CHARGE syndrome.

51. Consider "fever" among diseases -- in some situations?

52. Hawkins J., Op cit pp7-18/1-13

53. Sometimes called "heuristic."

54. Burch, H.B., JAMA, 2015;314(23): "Management of Graves Disease A Review" pp2544-2254

55. Orlander P., Medscape (Oct 14, 2016) "Toxic Nodular Goiter Clinical Presentation" 1/1

56. Loriaux L., John Wiley & Sons, Ltd. (2016) DOI: 10.1002/978119205791.ch58 "A Biographical History of Endocrinology+ 2/2

57. Sheridan, DJ., Imperial College Press London UK (2016) "Evidence-Based Medicine, Best Practice or Restrictive Dogma" pp192-193 and passim

58. Potts M., et al, BMJ (2006) September 30;333(7670), "Parachute approach to evidence based medicine" pp701-703

59. Hannan, SA., International Journal of Surgery. Volume 4, Issue 3, 2006 "The magnificent seven: a history of modern thyroid surgery" pp187-191

60. Dr. Theodor Billroth (1829-1894), Universities of Zurich and Vienna; and Dr. Theodor Kocher (1841-1917), who tried both total (result

as "cretinoid") and single lobectomy, gaining the name "Father of Thyroid Surgery."

61. Jayawardhana R., Scientific American/ Farrar, Straus, Giroux (2013) "Neutrino Hunters" pp3-210

62. Popper KR, Oxford University Press 1972 "Objective Knowledge" p9 and passim

63. Bird, R.M., Universities Libraries, Health Sciences Library, University of Oklahoma" Oklahoma City, Galileo and the Health Sciences Aug 7, 2015 – Apr 15, 2016 "A physician-engineer follower of Galileo applied the physics of the lever and other simple machines to the working of the musculoskeletal system." And, Galileo Galilei (1564-1642) Br J Sports Med 2006;40:806-807

64. These brief comments are found in several computer articles. One such is called "The History of Radiation" (https.//www.mirion/ introduction-to—radiation-safety/the-history-of radiation). Mme Curie is quoted to say science may be "…a benefit for mankind." She died of aplastic anemia.

65. Sheridan, DJ, Op cit pp 204-205 and passim

66. Sheridan, DJ, Ibid pp 204-205

67. Forstrom LA, The Journal of Medicine and Philosophy: A Forum for Bioethics and Philosophy of Medicine Volume 2, Issue 1, 1 January 1977 "The Scientific Autonomy of Clinical Medicine." pp8-19

68. Kuhn TS., Univ. of Chicago Press (1970) 2nd edition "The Structure of Scientific Revolutions" p15

69. Meinert CL, Op cit., p17 and passim

70. Hawkins, R., Op cit p2/13

71. Anscombe G.E.M., (posthumous), Edited by Feach M, and Gormally., Imprint Academic, UK(2015):: "And that a good many facts should be in such a position in our knowledge as to provide a framework into which everything else must fit…" p 187

72. Tannenbaum S., Academic Medicine Vol 74, Number 7 (1999), "Evidence and expertise: The challenge of the outcomes movement to medical professionalism" pp757-763

73. Bowen J, NEJM Number 23, 2006; 355: 2217-2225 "Educational Strategies to Promote Clinical Diagnostic Reasoning" passim

74. Norman G, Academic Medicine Volume 75 number 10., Oct Suppl., 2000" The epistemology of clinical reasoning: perspectives from philosophy, psychology, and neuroscience." 1999 Jack Maatsch Memorable Presentation pp S127-S133

75. Henty S., Theoretic Medicine and Bioethics 26:197 2006 "Recognizing Tacit Knowledge in Medical Epistemology" p188 and passim

76. Willis BH Family Practice 30:501-505, 1 July 2013 "Philosophy of science and the diagnostic process" Abstract and passim

77. Cohen AM International Journal of Medical Informatics, Volume 73, Issue 1, February 2004,"A categorization and analysis of the criticisms of Evidence-Based Medicine" pp 35-43

78. Knottnorus JA, BMJ Feb 23 2002 "Evaluation of diagnostic procedures: pp 477-480

79. Feinstein, AR, American Journal of Medicine Volume 103, Issue 6, December 1997 "Problems in the 'Evidence' of 'Evidence-Based Medicine'" pp 529-535

80. Lau J, BMJ 2006 Sep 16; 333(7568):597-600 "The case of the misleading funnel plot" passim

81. Tonelli, MR, Acad Med 1999 Nov 74(11): "In defense expert opinion" pp1187-92 (Abstract)

82. Meinert CL, Op Cit., Writing of randomized trials: "Likewise, there is no trial without money to do it. The money here comes from sponsors – generally, a drug company, foundation or governmental agency," p23

83. Every-Palmer S., Journal of Evaluation in Clinical Practice ISSN 1365-2753 (2014) "How evidence-based medicine is failing due to biased trials and selective publication" passim

84. Greenhalgh T, BMJ 348:g3725, 2014 Jun 13 "Evidence based medicine: a movement in crisis" passim

85. Wolpe PR, Sci Med (1990) 31:8, "Biomedical heresy is a form of science heresy..." p913

86. Meinert CL, Ibid., p27

87. Knottnerus JA, 2002 BMJ Feb 23; 324(7325): 477-480 Evidence base of clinical diagnosis, "Evaluation of diagnostic procedures" p478

88. Greenhalph T, BMJ 2014; 348: g3725. Published online 2014 Jun 13, doi:10:1136/bmj:g3725 Essay "Evidence based medicine: a movement in crisis?" p2/13 and passim

89. Every-Palmer S, Published online June 2014 DOI; 10:1111/ep:12147Source: PubMed "How evidence-based medicine is failing due to biased trials and selective publication" Abstract

90. Boyd C., JAMA, August 10, 2005 – volume 294, number 6 "Clinical Practice Guidelines and Quality of care for Older Patients with Multiple Comorbid Diseases." pp716-717

91. Meinert CL, Oxford University Press Inc. 2011 New York, New York "An insider's guide to clinical trials" p 60

92. Meinert CL, Ibid. Another quotation: "Hints at answers to the question of who pays for the trials can be gleaned from indexing (introduced in 2005) relating to support. As of October 14, 2010, there were 18,155 trials indexed to the publication type 'randomized controlled trials,' published in 2009 (English language and limited to human trials). Out of these, 2773 were funded in part of or totally by the US Public health service (mostly national institutes of health funding). The number of reports not listing any US government support was 8,716." p61

93. Meinert, CL., Ibid., p58

94. Fuzzy boundaries might interfere at times, but is usually dealt with repeat or other tests. Or such situations might lead to investigation and new knowledge.

95. Sheridan, DJ, Op cit., pp204-205 and passim

CHAPTER 9

Heritage: Times and medical science

Antiquity

Traditional methods of medical diagnosis reach far back in history, at least to what we know about cultures in ancient ages. These methods incorporate a fundamental quality of human beings, namely that certain causes bring about certain effects. It is true that science in ancient times would have been relatively primitive, whereas it would be false to believe that people had no causal explanations, but had many different ones. Nonetheless, Hippocrates (Greek, c. 460 – 370 BC), has been quoted thus: "He knew the cause of every malady." He created the Hippocratic Oath and has been called the Father of Medicine.[1] Some of his theory (four humors) is thought to be followed by Galen (Greek, 129–216 AD, anatomist and philosopher), who is believed to have partially modified the Hippocratic theory of humors. An anatomist, Galen investigated several bodily organs, and "the rest of the body through separate channels, nerves, arteries and veins." These early scientific medical studies of the human body and accompanying theories spread to languages through other civilizations. Influence of ancient Greek medicine is found in our world today.[1]

Interestingly, an article appeared recently in the New York Times, titled "'Organ' is found." Briefly, on the issue of a "'highway of moving fluid' and 'previously unknown feature of human anatomy.'" And, "We have never understood the mechanism of how that happens, said Dr. Neil Theise, a pathologist and professor at the New York University School of Medicine and a senior author on the paper."[2] This finding will be further investigated and may be of significant benefit to patients, if not now perhaps later along with newer knowledge. At least this new finding and theory hark back to the concepts, findings, and theories of the scientific accomplishments of ancient Greece.

The Middle Ages

During the Middle Ages, little new medical science is known, but some Greek influence continued for several (likely more) centuries. On another side, Ms. Cristina Millan writes, "The most famous and the most influential in European universities was the Canon of Medicine by Ibn Sina (Avicenna; 980 – 1037 A.D.)" from Islamic medicine. Ms. Millan describes several other medical contributions from Islamic physicians during this period, including new knowledge of parts of skeletal bones, function of the cardiac septum, and details of measles and smallpox.[3]

The Early Modern

The enterprising medical scientists in the middle and late nineteenth century followed their predecessors with growing investigations. The theory of germ diseases is an important example. Having long theoretical roots, the theory eventually became well established, yet continues to change and expand. The theory of disease by germs can also be found earlier among Islamic medical scientists (Ibn Sina, 980–1037, and Girolamo Fracastoro, 1478–1555). "Fracastoro proposed that diseases could spread in many ways—directly, indirectly or remotely. His 'seeds' or 'seedlets' could be chemical or living, and arose from sick bodies, spontaneously in the air or in decomposing matter."[4]

The progress in medical science during the nineteenth century led to even wider and deeper medical science in the early twentieth century. As previously discussed, Desmond Sheridan, in his new book *Evidence-Based Medicine*, writes of "the great strides made in the early twentieth century to introduce science into clinical settings" and "its retreat back to the laboratory is surely one of the great tragedies to befall medicine in the UK in recent decades" (Cf. Chapter 8). These two quotations come from changing methodological contexts (e.g., models), with mostly similar changes between the UK and other modern countries.

The innovations of medical science in early twentieth century were not alone. Dr. Richard C. Cabot created medicine curricula as a clinician and educator working at Harvard and Massachusetts General Hospital. He had a vibrant interest in his patient cases, including social ethics for them, patient diagnosis, and particularly the use of differential diagnoses. "He expanded the latter book to include the rest of the body, writing twelve editions from 1901 to 1938. His book, Differential Diagnosis, published in 1938, went through seven editions. He emphasized errors of omission and commission in clinical diagnosis."[5] The last sentence is best interpreted by the terms as test results counted "confirmatory" and/or "disconfirmatory" (Chapter 7).

Dr. Cabot formulated the list of differential diagnoses and the logical use of *confirmatory and disconfirmatory* in testing. The clinician gathers evidence by the patient's story (signs and symptoms, questions and answers), physical examination, relevant tests, and all are important. These methods became the traditional model for medical diagnosis through the remainder the twentieth century, and still, at least in modern western nations. If so, why this book? Well, a century after Dr. Cabot, and much other discussion in between, some reviews, changes, and additions should be warranted.

The Contemporary

Computers in the past few decades have brought large storage and access to information, changing many uses and habits in ordinary activities, including medical science and other sciences. In medicine, computers have made it possible to create three-dimensional images from internal human anatomy and videos of moving structures using computer tomography (CT). Similar technology has been used in other modalities, including MRI, PET, Ultrasound, etc. (Chapter 1). Most everyone will know that computers are involved in practically every aspect of information today, and surely in medicine. Nonetheless, however, clinicians are commonly busier than ever, managing loads of information. Computer assisted tests (e.g., MRI, PET, ECHO) add information of two kinds, the first being appropriate and successful in application, and the second being consequential of the test results, namely (if useful), depending on results being confirmatory or disconfirmatory, changing up or down probabilities of differential diagnoses. Such tests are beneficial, but may not offer a definitive diagnosis, for example if another test (e.g., a biopsy) is needed. The hardware is a worker, the scientist clinician a judge.

The Present and Future

Present

To some degree, new kinds of future medicine have been tried among us for a few decades. Some of these kinds (or hybrids) will be mentioned. All attempt to make diagnoses faster and cheaper, generally by using short-cuts.

Diagnostic EBM: This diagnostic model has marked short cuts and shortcomings, especially in patients with complicated diseases, and it has built in weaknesses for growth in medical science (Chapter 8).

Corporate medical care organizations (etc.): The title is ambiguous, covering many organizations. Their differences generally converge regarding the use of short cuts.

Hospitals and clinics (I): Addition of low-level technologies, e.g., computers and automated communication devices, displacing working people. Programs installed in such machines tend to be replaced frequently, as are the machines, as well as repairs for breakdowns and regular maintenance. I'm not an economist, yet one might wonder where short cuts lead.

Hospitals and clinics: Addition of high-level technologies, e.g., MRI, PET, ECHO, etc.

Lee A Forstrom

Hospitals and clinics – information (I) and (II):

(I)   Store and spread information:

Addition of low-level technologies, e.g., some computers
and automated communication devices may work differently.
Programs installed in such machines tend to be changed now
and then, and likely their programs more frequently. New
programs usually need training of operators. Maintenance
and breakdowns call for care. Guarding information security
calls for professionals. Perhaps these low-level technologies
are fully worth their time and costs for managers, clinicians, and patients, or they might also add to the pressure of
short cuts.

(II) Creation of new information:

Some will point out that these machines commonly need
computer assistance (e.g., MRI). That is true, but the technology levels of these imaging machines incorporate much
larger scientific matters. PET imaging, for example, blends
physics, chemistry, radiation, molecular metabolism, physiology, anatomy, and more—a machine with a computer. Such
images of internal structures and function generally provide
new and valuable information, with remarkable images and
established theory. Such pictures and videos are not "true
observables" (Cf. surgeons or pathologists), however, they
are high-level evidence. This would change the probabilities
of relevant differential diagnoses. Might this clash with
short cuts?

The Future

"Prediction is very difficult, especially if it's about the future."

Niels Bohr, Danish physicist, Nobel laureate (1885-1962) [6]

Niels Bohr theorized the structure of unobservable atoms as being analogous with our solar system. Similar with the planets moving in stable orbits around the sun, electrons must move in certain orbits around the positive charged nucleus. Like the planets, the electrons ordinarily follow stable orbits. If an electron orbit is unstable, for example struck by a foreign object, the shuffle of the electrons causes the atom to emit radiation. Remarkably, this source of radiation has played a fundamental role in medical radiology (Cf. Mme Curie et al, Chapter 8).

This example is the use of other sciences in scientific medicine. The discovery of radiation occurred about a century ago, a time span in which there has been great progress in science. Again, sciences are not fully separate, but rather share scientific information (e.g., physical chemistry).

This said, I prefer to abide with the wisdom from Niels Bohr.[6,7] Indeed, there are plenty of "safe" predictions, generally in common knowledge, such as big meteors and climate changes. My view of scientific medicine and its future can be found above (Chapter 8). Instead of predictions, there are a few current flaws and hopes for a better future that I will mention.

1. Hypotheses-Inferential (H-I) should be better than Hypothesis-deductive (H-D) as models for use in differential diagnosis. H-D has been a dominant model for at least a century. H-I has been refined in this treatise, however, by better accommodation of both logic and probabilities.

2. Another diagnostic model, Evidence-based Medicine (EBM), has been tried in about thirty years. This model ignores medical theory and relevant mechanisms, depending on statistics and rigid rules. The first suspicious diagnosis, followed by the first test showing confirmatory result (if done), is likely to be accepted. Other possible diagnoses, including risky ones, are likely dismissed. This method is simply too skimpy in clinical work, especially dealing with complex diseases. Since more thorough in managing simple as well as complex patient conditions by better models, like those above (H-I/H-D), there seems to be little need for EBM.

3. Haste is a problem for both clinicians and patients. This has been a complaint for a long time, but now seems worse. I have no numbers for this, but I have been on both sides for experience. In fact, I feel less pampered. I know patients who wait for days—or much longer—to see their doctor for fifteen minutes. They say that their doctor uses about half of the fifteen minutes looking into her/his computer. Not long ago, my wife and I both received a regular interview and examination, with follow up for any additional care.

4. A business model. This seems to be necessary for audits to stay in the black for present medical care, at least in our country. Hospitals, and particularly clinics, have grown like mushrooms, pretty and full with newness. But both clinicians and patients are likely more anxious than in older times. Both sides are prone to worry about the short visits and the high costs. For the clinician, many of the costs come from digital technology, devices, and upgrades, along with routine maintenance. Patients are likely to be concerned about their insurance, and to some degree the clinicians.[7] But the largest concern for the patient should be the compressed time with the clinician, especially making diagnoses.

The relevant clinician should be the best judge of diagnoses, after satisfactory interview and examination, and in nearly all cases needs time for analytical reasoning.[8,9]

5. Medical insurance applies to most everyone. Again, I have no numbers, but have some experience. I will mention only two issues.

> First: Clinicians pay for insurance to cover a possible mistake in caring of a patient. This could involve diagnosis or treatment, or both. Clinicians in some places, using the EBM model and following strict rules and statistics, might change the legalities, and perhaps also the business model (my conjecture).

> Second: The wide majority of people in our country have medical insurance, and most are glad for it, but a significant minority have minimal or no medical insurance, unlike most other modern nations. This issue should be seen as a matter of ethics and morality. Beauchamp and Childress illuminate many theories and fine points, but on this point write, "Countries lacking a comprehensive and coherent system of health care financing and delivery are destined to continue on the trail of higher costs and large numbers of unprotected citizens."[10] These authors follow with, "Policies of just access to health care, strategies of efficiency in health care institutions, and global needs for the reduction of health-impairing conditions dwarf in social importance every other issue considered in this book."[11] The first quotation applies to countries in general—and seems reasonably fit for our country. The issue here is that of ethics and morality. Our society should do better at home, and when feasible try to help global needs for better health on our planet.

6. Human genomes: The world of medicine changed on April 14, 2003, with the announcement of the "successful completion of the Human Genome Project."[12] Most physicians and many others were astounded, and most still are. The numbers are amazing, thus: "The human genome contain approximately 3 billion of these base pairs, which reside in the 23 pairs of chromosomes within the nucleus of all our cells. Each chromosome contains hundreds to thousands of genes, which carry the instructions for making proteins. Each of the estimated 30,000 genes in the human genome makes an average of three proteins."[13] Not surprisingly, physicians work for new discoveries between genes and diseases. While statistical correlations can be helpful, along with relevant medical knowledge, more investigation is needed for establishing causal connections. Those connections require further investigation to be accepted as sound. Modifier genes may affect the primary gene. This fits well in use of tendency laws, as discussed via sickle cell anemia earlier (Chapter 4). Unravelling the connections with other diseases will take time. Along with research physicians, clinicians in the field will also be heard.

Conclusion:

A leading purpose of this book has been an account of science and logic in medical diagnosis. In uncovering the roots of these subjects, we gain understanding in both analysis and structure used in dominant methods of medical diagnosis. Moreover, it has become clear to our predecessors that medicine is best as a science. Like other sciences, medical science stands on theory. That this theory changes and grows as it is recurrently put to the test of experience, in ordinary clinical contexts, in what has been an underlying theme in this account, that modern clinical medicine enjoys a vigorous scientific status. Few other sciences are applied and investigative activities so closely and of practical necessity interwoven.

Clinical medicine shares a variety of problems in common with other sciences -- it is not wholly typical or lacking in special methods. It holds, for obvious reasons, singular importance to the <u>individual patient</u>. This brings up an important issue with the methodological shortcomings in such cases, if given only statistical approaches (e.g., EBM). Another method, however, is available and fits with a traditional diagnostic model (H-D). A similar model was outlined in this book (H-I), being more complete and accurate. Compared to the first model above (EBM), both latter models deliver more evidence, including many known scientific mechanisms, established theories, clinical experience, subjective probabilities, and context. All of these are contained in the clinician's medical knowledge, generally with additional questions and patient exams in building an initial list of differential diagnoses.

Advocates of clinical models would favor psychological kinds of reasoning in diagnosis. The most accepted version has only two kinds, one a short cut mental grasp of a thing. Quick thinking should apply to a first impression, for example an observable injury, or perhaps a pattern recognition. A second kind of reasoning would be analytical, taking more time to think. This kind of reasoning would involve a deeper level of understanding, usually needed by the clinician to create the differential diagnoses in patients with difficult, complex, or multiple conditions. The EBM clinician, however, shuns many of the channels mentioned above, commonly ignoring such evidence not included in rigid rules. Moreover, the reference standard is used to select a possible diagnosis, based essentially on manifestations—some sort of aligning with other patients. Seemingly, a reference standard would be limited in both scope and depth, thus diminishing use in patients with common and complex diseases.

Two Points

First: The matter of unique patients

This matter was raised at the end of the previous chapter (Chapter 8) and brushed again in the matter of human genomes in this chapter. It is well known that the genome of any particular human subject is unique, making the person also unique. Differences acquired in life's journeys add to those at birth, expanding singularities between identical twins. True, statistical correlations can draw attention, but medical science is needed to find and establish causal linkages between genes and targets. In my perspective, in the long run, the latter should be the winner: discovering new diseases and treatments, perhaps helping even some very unique patients.

Second: Complex humans

Most clinicians are busy working with patients. A few, however, work at times to make better digital devices or programs. I have mentioned powerful computers working in body imaging, and other uses, saving many patients from worsening disease. In the hands of clinicians and technicians, computer programs trend to algorithms, again using rules (Chapter 8). However, for most work and play, less cost, and more security (privacy), humans are still ahead of machines, including computers. In fact, given human brains, my view is that human beings are the most complex and charming of all entities in the known universe. We should show such respect for individual patients, along with most all other persons.

REFERENCES AND FOOTNOTES: CHAPTER 9

1. Nutton V., edit., Bynam, W. and H., Great Discoveries in Medicine, 2011, Thames and Hudson LTD, London "Humours and Pneumas: The Hippocratic tradition." Hippocrates' son-in-law, Polybus, is said to have contributed. pp26-29

2. Fortin J., New York Times "Organ' is found" Re-published in Star Tribune, Minneapolis MN, SH2, April 15, 2018.

3. Millan C. A., edit., Bynam, W. and H.,Op cit., "Islamic Medicine,"pp30-33, and Abu Marwan Ibu Zuhr, 12th century; "The art of Medicine is based on the assessment of the practical experience." p31

4. Nutton V., edit., Op cit. : Worboys, M., "Germs – The greatest medical discovery" p69 This quotation goes on: "His ideas had little impact until his elevation as a precursor of germ theories in the late 19th century." p69

5. Croskerry P., The American Journal of Medicine (2008) Vol 121 (5A) S24-S29 "Overconfidence in Clinical Decision Making" S25

6. Ellis AK, Quoted in Teaching and Learning Elementary Social Studies (1970), Wikipedia

7. Bohr N., Philos. Mag. 26, 1 (1913) "The Constitution of Atoms and Molecules." pp 1-24

8. Groopman J., Op cit., p8

9. Gil C., Op cit., p1080

10. Beauchamp T.l., and Childress J.F., Op cit., p293

11. Beauchamp T.l., and Childress J.F., Ibid p293

12. https://www.genome.gov/11006943/ National Human Genome Research Institute, NIH, U.S. Department of Energy, October 30, 2010 p1/7

13. Ibid p1/7

Index

www.ingramcontent.com/pod-product-compliance
Lightning Source LLC
Chambersburg PA
CBHW020859180526
45163CB00007B/2563